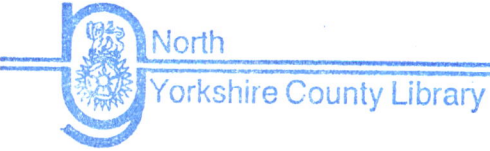

Some Yorkshire Bridges
of Beauty and Romance

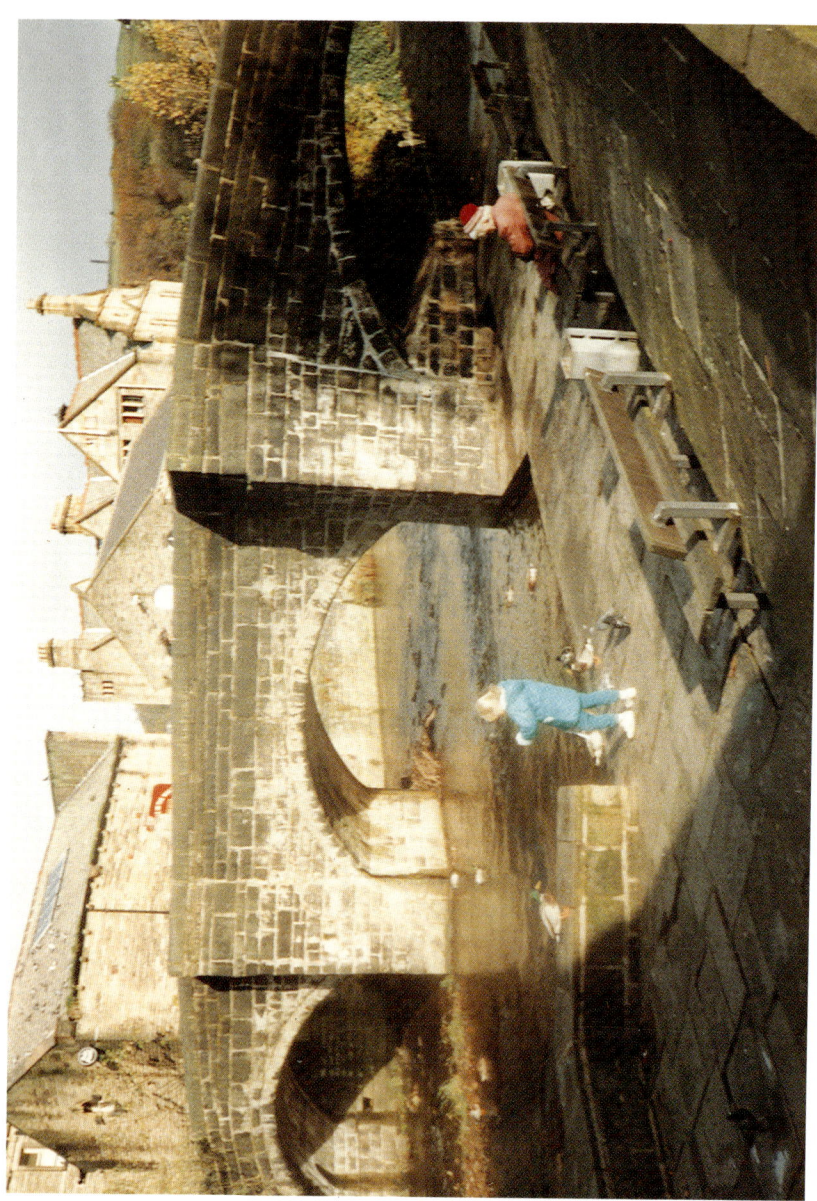

Hebden Packhorse Bridge

Some YORKSHIRE BRIDGES
of Beauty and Romance

Arnold N Patchett

The Pentland Press Limited
Edinburgh · Cambridge · Durham

First published in 1992 by
The Pentland Press Ltd.
5 Hutton Close
South Church
Durham

ISBN 1   872795   86   2

Jacket watercolour by Ruth Patchett
Typeset by Elite Typesetting Techniques,
Southampton.
Printed and bound by Antony Rowe Ltd.,
Chippenham.

ACKNOWLEDGEMENTS

Whilst much of the text of this book results from very many years of personal observation and local enquiry, the works of the following have been consulted, especially for exact dates:

Geoffrey Wright and Susan Cunliffe-Lister
and
the late Dr TD Whitaker, Rev Bailey Harker
Edmund Bogg, Harry Speight, Ella Pontefract and E Jervoise

More recently, the following have been of assistance in various ways:

Dr DA Hodgson and Mr Philip Rushworth of Bradford
Mr John Wright of Grassington
Rev SGN Brindley of Rotherham
Mrs Dorothy Jackson of Green Hammerton
Mr John Barnes of Skip Bridge
Mr P Young of Ossett, Wakefield
The staff of Castleford Public Library

CONTENTS

The following are the rivers or valleys where the bridges mentioned in the text are to be seen:

LIST OF ILLUSTRATIONS

†Photo: CA Brough   *Photo: the author

INTRODUCTION

In a letter to a Canadian newspaper during the Blitz on London in World War II, the following appeared:

> Be it said to your renown
> That you wore your gayest gown
> Your bravest smile, and stayed in town
> While London Bridge was falling down.

It referred, of course, to the Queen Mother, as Queen, when she said that she was glad that Buckingham Palace had been bombed. It made her feel that she and the King could look the East End in the face.

Very many other things fell down at that time, but a bridge was chosen by the author of that couplet. Bridges must surely possess some magic. So much so that London Bridge (built in 1831) was greatly desired in the USA. This historic structure across the Thames, having become inadequate to cope with increasingly heavy traffic and being offered for sale, was snapped up for $2,460,000 by developers of Lake Havasu City on the Colorado River. Stone by numbered stone was transported across the Atlantic and then across the USA, and rebuilt over an arm of the lake at a cost of a further $5,600,000! Just to add a little colour to the scene, a red English telephone booth was placed near the site and by a seat overlooking the water.

Europe especially possesses very many bridges, both ancient and modern. The mind flits from the Bridge of Sighs in Venice to the magnificent river crossing of the Danube at Budapest, the Pont du Gard in France, and, nearer home, the Pulteney Bridge in Bath. With the bridge at Stamford Bridge in Yorkshire in mind, I am led to have a close look at some of

Yorkshire's bridges. In this book, I am ignoring some of the new boundaries which have robbed parts of:

> Bonnie Yorkshire and all that she enfolds
> From the Humber to the Tees
> From the Pennines to the Wolds
> . . . . . .

In these days of concrete and steel 'architecture', we are now beginning to
look more carefully than ever at the sheer beauty and indeed workmanship
of our heritage of bridges, of which there are so many in Yorkshire. Some
suffer because they happen to be on our way to beauty spots, and, in our
haste to reach our objective, we hardly notice them. Others are often
ignored because they are in industrial or semi-industrial areas, but are
nonetheless full of interest. The bridges at Wakefield, Hebden Bridge,
Ripponden and Rotherham are good examples. Wakefield and Rotherham
both have a chantry chapel integral with the bridge and date back far into
the past.

I allow myself to be side-tracked from time to time to discover a little gem
hidden away from the average tourist routes.

In the case of places like York, Knaresborough and Richmond, the
history of these towns is inseparable from the bridges they possess. Much
has already been written about them by others, but we cannot possibly pass
them by without some reference.

I trust the reader will forgive me for omitting reference to one or more of
his favourite bridges. I am sure that there are many which warrant some
mention, but sufficient for the day . . .

ANP

STAMFORD BRIDGE

Stamford Bridge, or Pons Belli as it was often called, was of course the scene of the actual battle of that name in AD 1066.

King Harold's alienated brother, Tostig, and the King of Norway, Hardrada, joined forces to lay claim to at least part of England. To this end they sailed up the Humber, the Ouse and then the Derwent, but on reaching Stamford Bridge were routed by Harold, Tostig being killed.

Unfortunately, a 'second front' against Harold in the form of an invasion came about at Pevensey in Sussex. Harold took all he could muster from his victorious army and went to meet the invader, William of Normandy. We all know the result of the Battle of Hastings, but the memory of the victory at Stamford Bridge lingers on, in spite of the former which completely altered the course of English history.

The bridge at Stamford appears to have been built of timber, most likely on stone piers, and is said to have stood some 50 yards upstream from the present structure. In 1727, "a high and narrow bridge with three arches was built and is likely to be the one which is now in use. The width between the parapets is 13 feet except over one arch which has been widened by about six feet". Because of this, the niches at that particular end have disappeared, only the two at the other end remaining. All three arches are segmental. The bridge was mentioned in medieval records and wills, and in 1282, an order was made to pay the sum of £20 to Robert, Rector of Sutton-on-Derwent, for its repair. This must have been in respect of the original bridge upstream.

Today the bridge is still narrow, and one-way traffic is the order of the day, with traffic lights at each end. There are iron stays, the ends of which show under the parapets, and on the upstream side a large pipe spans the water, as well as a walkway. Fortunately these can only been seen at fairly close quarters and are almost hidden from the banks on the downstream side, except of course, for the iron stays. The old jetties are still there and serve as a reminder of the former frequent river traffic.

Stamford Bridge is a popular stopping place, with hostelries on both sides of the river which date back many years. One is the Three Cups, which is built on a well. In fact, the modern bar counter lies over it which enables visitors to view the depths through a circular opening. To aid viewing, the well is illuminated. The inn was quite undeveloped up until the 1960s when the then owners, Mr & Mrs Wilson Lee, beautifully restored it. Further improvements have since been made. Upstream, a little way from the bridge, is the huge five-storied corn mill complete with water wheel, which dominates the scene in a most pleasant way. It is now a commodious inn with a great variety of public rooms, including the Wheel Bar.

DOWN SWALEDALE AND ITS BRIDGES

Great Sleddale Beck, Little Sleddale Beck and Birkdale Beck are sizeable headwaters of the Swale, and at Hoggarth's Bridge – often called High Bridge – we join the Swale proper, typical of the many in this vast gathering ground, rugged and strong. To see a lovely little packhorse affair with a single arch and parapets, one has to trek up Whitsundale Beck to Raven Seat, a tiny and quite remote hamlet which was, some 250 years ago, a thriving spot sporting an inn. Packhorses could then be seen carrying their loads, chiefly coal, over that sturdy little crossing.

Back to the Swale again to find Low Bridge which leads to Smithy House, but before we part company with the main road, it is worth mentioning that there are many signs marked 'C to C' (Coast to Coast Path) in and around Swaledale. There is one just north-east of Birkdale Cross, the latter being on the main road to Kirkby Stephen.

Passing Park Bridge on our left, we turn left and slip into Keld village. We forsake bridges for a while to follow the Swale's spectacular course down the valley, both north and south of Keld, to look at Catrake Foss and Kisdon Foss, waterfalls the like of which one never sees again along the river's course to Catterick and beyond to Myton, the Ure and the Ouse.

Returning to the main road again, leaving the Swale to hide itself behind Kisdon as it courses through a very steep-sided valley, we come to Thwaite with its attractive little bridge over its beck. Thwaite was the birthplace of the brothers Richard and Cherry Kearton who made a great study of the district and became well known naturalists. Over the bridge we go and before reaching Muker cross yet another one.

The bridge at Muker itself has one arch, seemingly old enough to have been there since the beginning of time, which enables us to cross the Muker Beck on our way down the dale, and the view of it from downstream, somewhat shrouded with small trees and bushes, with the background consisting of the church tower and some of the village, is one which artists have painted times without number. The church, whilst ancient enough and rugged, has stood there only since 1580, after Leland's time. To join the Swale, we have to go downstream a little distance.

But the bridge of bridges only a few miles east of Muker must surely be that of Ivelet. It is a single-arched structure less than half the width of that at Muker, and in the middle almost twice as high. It is in fact a packhorse bridge and loads were carried in panniers slung over the animals' heads, much of the trade in Upper Swaledale passing this way. Tales of Bargest, the legendary dog of the Yorkshire Dales, which had no master, are

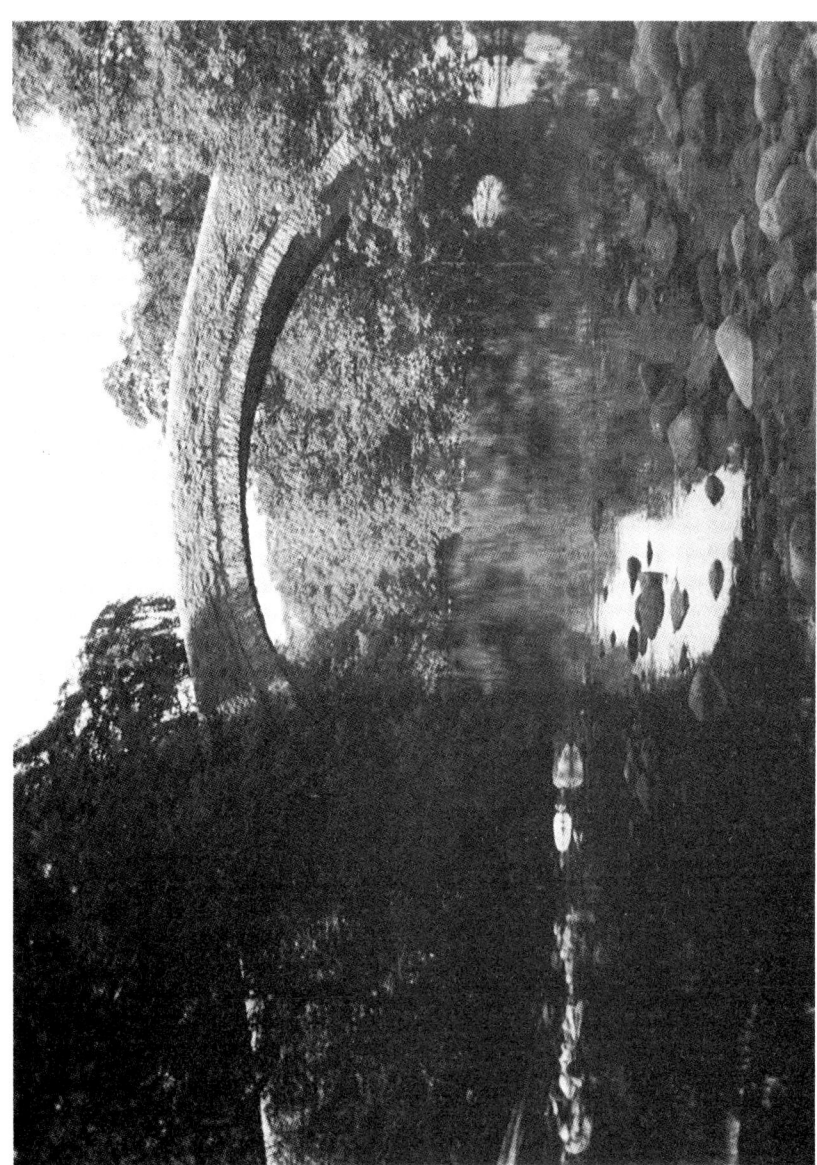

Ivelet Bridge

associated with Ivelet Bridge. For sheer symmetry and beauty, the bridge has few, if any, equals. Known as the Humpbacked Bridge, it is still used by modestly-sized farm vehicles and to see it at its best one should view it midmorning looking upstream. If the river is smooth-surfaced, as it often is at this point, one is rewarded with a superb reflection mirroring the wonderful and skilful workmanship of the builders of so long ago. To complete the picture, a splashing beck joins the Swale just before the latter passes under the bridge.

The lane from the main road down the dale leads to the bridge quite sharply and crosses the water to the hamlet of Ivelet, and is believed to have been part of the Corpse Way – a long track from the upper reaches of the Swale to Grinton and its church. The dead were carried in wicker baskets by bearers across Ivelet Bridge to Grinton until the church at Muker was built.

Bridge after bridge crosses and recrosses the river before it reaches that gem of the north country – Richmond.

From Ivelet there is an unusual bridge which crosses the river to Gunnerside. It has two almost semicircular arches with very low cutwaters and a level carriageway, quite wide, and it, too, forms a lovely picture in the morning sunshine. It is called New Bridge and enables the traveller to follow the main road to Reeth and across the Swale to Grinton. As well as Swale Hall, a romantic residence, now a farm, Grinton possesses a very ancient church – "The Cathedral of the Dales" – which was, as previously mentioned, the end of the Corpse Way. A few miles further on, we leave the main road and cross the river yet again to join the old road from Richmond up the dale, by means of another, quite unusual, very high bridge with two huge arches, with the carriageway built on a marked incline to the north. In a short while we reach that little jewel of a village – Marske.

Marske is set in one of the most beautiful parts of Swaledale. It stands near the swift-flowing rivulet, Marske Beck, in a well-wooded area; a great variety of trees was planted by the Hutton family who became owners of the manor in the late 16th century. The first was Matthew Hutton who, at that time, was Archbishop of York. One of his descendants, another Matthew, also became Archbishop. There are spectacular views of the white cliffs crowning the steep and well-wooded south bank of the Swale.

Markse Bridge is one which crosses the beck, and the best view of it is from the grounds of Marske Hall. It dates from the 15th century and shows the old stonework where it integrates with the rocky bank. It consists of a single arch and parapet on both sides, and has chamfered ribs supporting it on the downstream side to the extent of two-thirds. The remaining third of the arch is comparatively modern and, though integrated with the old, is lower by a few inches than the latter. Up to about two-thirty in the afternoon, the downstream side can be delightfully lit up with sunshine without interference from trees, and the trees upstream form a colourful backcloth in early autumn.

The builders of this most attractive crossing certainly had an eye for symmetry and grace. Repairs in 1588 are said to have cost £25, and a further £20 had to be spent about a hundred years later. It saw packhorses with their loads on their way to and from Richmond and to Downholme on their way to Wensleydale. Their route would, no doubt, pass by Walburn Hall, a quite remarkable Elizabethan manor house, with traces of Norman work in one of the walls suggesting an earlier house belonging to the Walburn family. One of them, Wymer de Walburn, held a number of oxgangs of land there in 1286. The Hall is about midway between Marske and Leyburn.

On the way to Richmond, one of the finest towns in England, by the old road from Marske, a path leads to Willance's Leap. William Willance, a wealthy man from Richmond, was out hunting on his horse and suddenly met with fog. The horse leaped into the deep ravine, but Willance fell off and got away with a broken leg. Three stones were erected to commemorate his escape through God's grace.

And so we enter Richmond, with its splendid castle ruins, the view from which is truly magnificent. The castle, largely 12th century, surmounts the sheer cliffs straight up from the river. To the north of the castle is Greyfriars Tower, all that remains of the Franciscan Friary of 1258.

Eighteenth century Frenchgate is a steep and narrow hard northern edition of Gold Street in Shaftesbury, but has more houses. Portergate, Callowgate, Bargate to name but a few are typical of this unique town. A huge market place, once surrounded largely by very good houses, now mostly shops, contains Holy Trinity Church, part of which now houses the Green Howards Museum. Also standing there is a tall obelisk dated 1771 on the site of the one-time market cross. Before we go down to the river by means of Bargate, we must slip out of the Square and have a look at the restored Georgian Theatre Royal, 1788, now possibly the best example of such a theatre in the whole of England. The proscenium is almost perfect. Ground-floor boxes are there as well as upper boxes supported on Tuscan columns. The pay box, stage, dressing rooms and staircase are original.

Richmond truly warrants a long stay in order to enjoy its many and varied attractions, so we reluctantly make our way down Bargate to have a look at the bridge which figures on so many views of 'Richmond from the river' on postcards, paintings and sketches.

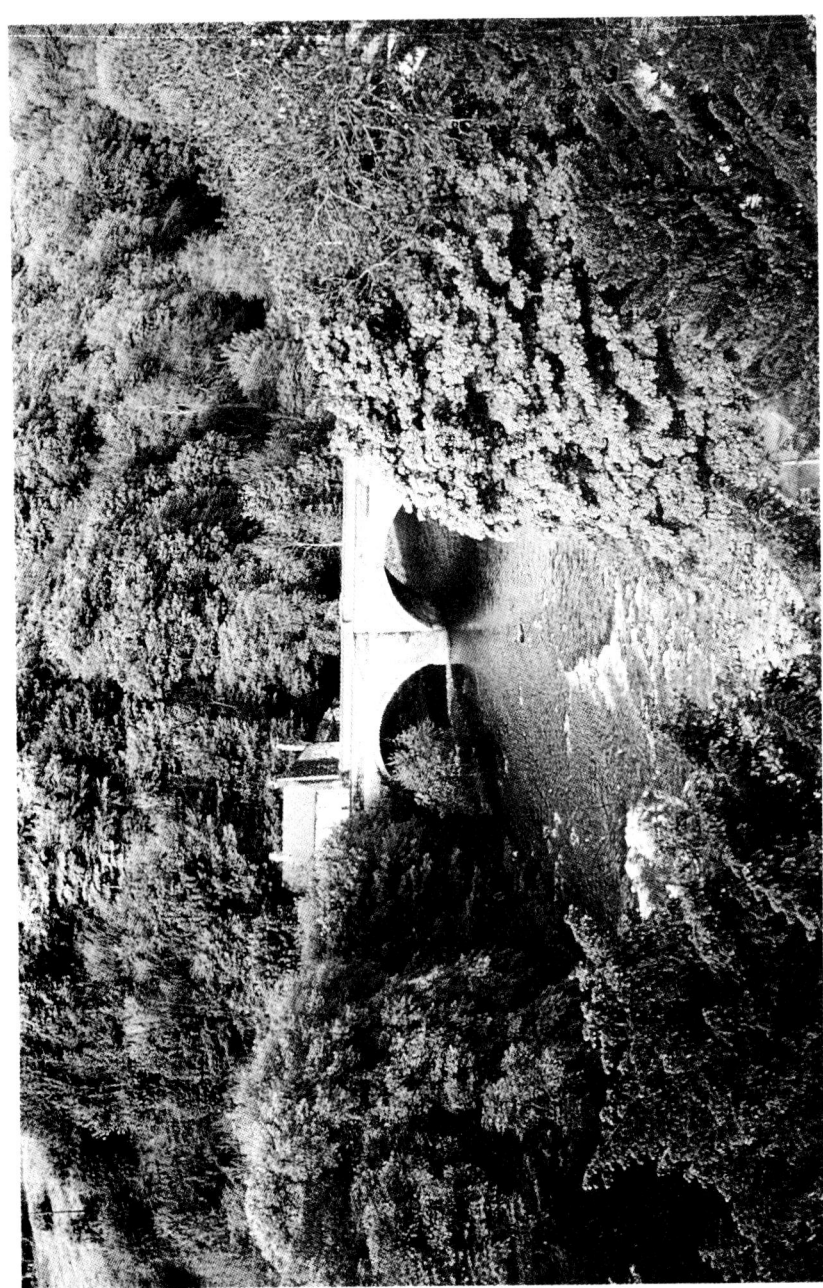

The bridge at Richmond

From whichever viewpoint we take, the bridge has charm. Looking down from the castle ramparts, one sees, far below, the crossing set in the middle of a prolific area of woodland with the silvery Swale gliding under the arches. From the narrow road at the foot of the beetling cliffs below the castle, there is an urge to hurry forward and turn sharply left to stand on the bridge and survey the attractive scene both up and down stream. Fortunately, most of the traffic to and from Richmond crosses the river lower down by means of a more modern bridge near the one-time railway station, and that which goes up the valley keeps to the north of the river for a time.

Crossing the river, then, by the old bridge leads to a path on the right and, in a few hundred yards, one arrives at the spot where so many artists and photographers stop for a while. The bridge has three graceful arches with semi-circular cutwaters and has the stamp of that great architect, John Carr, who was responsible for so many elegant structures, including bridges in York and the old North Riding. Rebuilding took place early in the 19th century when the bridge was widened, the width between parapets being increased to 27 feet.

Leland in his itinerary said it had four arches (16th century), and that great cartographer, Speed, agreed with this in 1610, but in October 1739, the Sessions discussed a contract for repairs. The emphasis is on the word 'discussed'!

The next bridge of special note must surely be Catterick.

Whilst Catterick village, and its bridge some one and a half miles to the north, are on the old Great North Road, they are both east of the Roman road from Boroughbridge to Piercebridge. Curiously enough, the modern North Road leaves the old route about a mile south of the village and follows roughly the Roman road to Scotch Corner, crossing the Swale near to where the old wooden bridge once stood.

A stone bridge was built by private enterprise in the first half of the 15th century with three arches, but by 1575 it is said that it was to be rebuilt and the sum of £1750 was needed to do this. During the 17th century the north pier especially needed further expenditure and, in 1615, a John Johnson, plaisterer, was to undertake the work of keeping the bridge in repair over a period of seven years for a fee of £260. In spite of this, the cost by 1634 amounted to £588:4:8d. and even only 40 years later the bridge was described as 'very ruinous' – not by Leland this time! All the water pressure was exerted at the north end because a bank of sand at the south end had formed, so little or no water passed through that arch.

The present substantial bridge has four segmental arches and pointed cutwaters with sloping tops. It is a good-looking structure, but the medieval stonework is hidden by widening and new ashlar faces. The widening by 16 feet resulted in a carriageway of about 30 feet, sufficient for any amount of traffic. When one surveys the bridge today, the first thing that impresses one is its massive solidity, so it is not surprising that it has stood the test of time over so many years with the enormous amount of traffic of all kinds, including railway locomotives and their wagons on rails when the military camp was first established; the railway traffic ceased, however, in 1922, when a steel bridge was erected to take the rails. In spite of the ceaseless traffic on the modern A1, Catterick Bridge still carries a surprisingly large number of vehicles of all kinds.

In between the old road and the new is the famous racecourse, but the village of Catterick lies over a mile to the south of its famous bridge. Less famous, but none the less attractive, are the three little bridges in and around the village itself. Coming from the south, then, one crosses the first over Catterick Beck, along the old North Road as it enters Catterick. The first left turn after this reveals the Angel Inn, an ancient coaching house. Keeping to the right of it, one is rewarded with a view of absolute charm. The beck, some ten to twelve feet wide, gurgles its way between well-kept grassy banks, and on each side there are some extremely interesting houses. Some are Georgian, some are earlier and some later, but all complement each other. Proceeding upstream one reaches the Bay Horse Inn and the Oak Tree Inn, as well as a large triangular green. Mature trees stand at intervals along the banks of the beck which is crossed by a little stone bridge near the Oak Tree. Water fowl quietly approach you and look for food, but if none is forthcoming they waddle away without complaint.

Special mention is needed of the house numbered 43, dated 1709. Its door and decorated bow windows give the place great charm. There are several others with lovely doorways and others with both doors and windows of special note.

The church of St Anne – well worth a visit – is approached up a steep and narrow side street, and a brief history is available for a small offering. Paulinus is said to have visited Catterick in the 7th century and baptised, in the Swale, throngs of people ready to be converted to Christianity. A window in the church shows Paulinus in the act of baptising.

We cross the beck once again by a pleasant footbridge and leave this lovely village to reach the hurly-burly of the old North Road, as we ruminate on Catterick's past. It was a centre for tanning from AD 80 to AD 120, leather being produced for footwear, tents and parts of soldier's uniforms. Romans, Anglo Saxons and Normans have all known Catterick, Cataractonium in Roman times. The George Inn, now the Bridge House

Hotel, was established as long ago as the 15th century, and was an important stopping place, as was The Angel in the village. The Bridge House is a long rambling place and, though modernised in many ways, still retains some of its old character.

The Roman camp was just over the river from the Hotel, on land now between the new and old Great North Roads.

PIERCEBRIDGE

From Catterick we can follow the Roman road, or at least most of it, on its way to Hadrian's Wall at Portgate. A mile or so from Scotch Corner, we turn left and shortly find ourselves on a long straight road, but as we approach the River Tees the road suddenly turns left, passes an ancient hostelry, The George, turns right and crosses over the river into Pierce-bridge village with its spacious green.

The bridge we have just crossed is described by our old friend, Leland, as 'Perse Bridge sumtime of 5 arches, but a late made new of 3 Arches'. What he said is still true, so we can assume that it was built no later than the early part of the 16th century, and to suit the traffic of that time, it was 13 feet wide.

Its ancient pointed arches, and the wee arch supporting the carriageway as it bends towards the west, are best seen from upstream in the early afternoon, especially when the sun is shining. The wee arch just referred to is itself supported partially by the northern half of the last of the pointed arches. Viewed from the garden of The George, the widened downstream side of the bridge is quite evident. The rounded arches and the line of demarcation between the old and the new is plainly visible on the underside of the arches.

If Leland found that the bridge was in a 'ruinous state' when he visited it, he didn't appear to make any comment on the matter. However, some 65 years later, after his death, it was reported in the Sessions of 1616 that the bridge was ruinous and decayed and that the responsibility for its repair was sought. Nothing much appears to have been done, for, in 1625, it was 'in great ruin especially on the Yorkshire side'. Twenty years later, it was stated as being broken down for a distance of 12 yards, the rest being in decay. The arches on the old (upstream) side show little signs of rebuilding, so it seems that it was the approaches and the carriageway which needed the bulk of attention. In any case, by 1673 it appears that all had been put to rights, but the bridge has been considerably widened on the downstream side since then.

Cutwaters right up to the top of the parapets enable foot passengers to indulge in the oft-found pleasure of leaning over the parapet without the fear of impeding vehicular traffic whilst also ensuring their own safety. And what lovely views there are to enjoy, both up and down stream.

In our haste to have a good look at the bridge and proceed further up the valley, we are apt to miss the site of the original one – the Roman crossing of the Tees. If, instead of bearing left on approaching the Tees, we continue almost in a straight line down a tiny lane, we come to the site of the Roman bridge. In comparatively recent times, excavations for gravel on the present south side of the river have revealed, amongst a great deal of stonework abutments, foundations of piers and part of the paved bed of the river. It appears that the Tees has slowly eroded the north bank, and left the south high and dry with vast quantities of gravel since Roman times. Nature has done the rest over the years by greening over the gravel silt and the stonework partially broken down by water, frost and other causes. So, for centuries, the gigantic blocks of stone bonded together with Roman mortar and metal clamps, together with the rest of the remains, have stood undetected, but are now open to the sky for all to see. Descriptive plaques in the area help one to visualize the bridge as it once stood. There is no admission charge.

Immediately across the river is the site of the Roman civil settlement, and, to the west of it, the military fort – Morbium. Having been excavated some years ago, detailed and photographed, the civil site is now fully restored to agriculture. To the west, the military fort is permanently exposed and maintained, and open to the public. It is approached from the village under which the remainder of the fort lies, presumably for all time. The north-east corner of the fort has been open to the sky for many years and is approached from the north of the village.

Now we can see why the modern road turns right after leaving the village. It joins the one-time Roman road, after it had crossed the Tees, on its way north to Hadrian's Wall.

Resisting the temptation to visit the famous bridge at Croft-on-Tees for the moment, let us go up river to Greta Bridge via Winston Bridge to join yet another Roman road on its way westward to Carlisle.

Winston Bridge consists of one gigantic and lofty arch spanning the Tees. The best view is from upstream – a path on the south side leads one to a pebble beach. The swift-flowing water passes over an anything but smooth river bed, and adds to the charm of the well-wooded steep sides of the valley.

A few miles takes us to the Scotch Corner – Penrith road where we turn right for Greta Bridge, Rokeby and Brignall.

GRETA BRIDGE

The nearby Morritt Arms at Rokeby, long since by-passed by the modern A66, much to the relief of patrons of the hotel endeavouring to sleep in the front bedrooms, is a natural stopping place.

The bridge is regarded by many as unique, in this part of England at any rate. It can be viewed from several points, and from each one derives great pleasure. It is difficult to imagine that, not so many years ago, it bore all the heavy traffic from the famous Scotch Corner to Carlisle. It was built in 1789, at a cost of £850, by Mr JBS Morritt, who inherited it from Mr John Sawrey Morritt, and was a friend of Sir Walter Scott, who, of course, wrote:

> O, Brignall banks are wild and fair
> And Greta woods are green,
> And you may gather garlands there
> Would grace a summer queen.

This is another bridge which bears the stamp of the architect, John Carr of York. The structure consists of one main and graceful segmental arch complete with balustraded parapets, and is 80 feet from end to end. There is a small arch at the western end which gives access from one pasture to another and provides a relief for flood waters. The condition at present is just about perfect – Leland, if he were alive today, could not fail to praise it. There are two piers, one at each end, which rise to the top of the parapets to provide niches; two paterae in the spandrels add a final touch to its beauty.

Again, we have a bridge much painted and photographed. No sooner had it been built when Thomas Girtin painted it. This artist, famous for his work in Yorkshire, displayed his gift in a picture of Kirkstall Abbey in 1799.

Leland, when he visited the bridge in the first half of the 16th century, described it as having 'two or three' arches. In 1552, ten years after his death, a great deal of money was spent on repairs. This went on for years in an endeavour to keep it sound, but in 1771 it was washed away in a great flood. There must have been a temporary structure pending completion of the present one.

The river is, of course, the Greta which, having flowed through Brignall, passes under the bridge on its way to the Tees. On following it, by means of a path starting just east of the gates of Rokeby Hall, one reaches the main river at Watersmeet.

At the west end of the bridge are the gates of the Hall; they are Grecian, and form a grand entrance with spacious greensward between them and the road leading to the Morritt Arms. In the hall of the hotel are relics of the Roman era when a fort was built here. It was largely on land at the back of the hotel, and the west boundary is marked by a lane leading to Brignall. Part of the stone facing of a rampart is visible near the one-time south gate of the fort, which occupied something like three and a half acres.

CROFT BRIDGE

Quite suddenly one arrives at Croft, the one-time spa. The Georgian Croft Spa Hotel, the ancient church and bridge form a most attractive trio.

The very important crossing of the Tees from the south to Darlington in days gone by, long before the bridge to the west at Blackwell was built, was at Croft. The Tees is much enlarged here through the waters of the Skerne entering it a little upstream from the bridge.

A bridge over the Tees at Croft was known in the 14th century because a grant of pontage was made in 1356 for its repair as it was, like so many, in a dangerous state following a great flood. One feels that during the 16th century Leland may well have reported to Henry VIII that part of the foundations of three of the piers had been washed away, again by flood waters, as repairs were carried out during the King's reign. Further repairs were made in 1570, some years after Leland's time.

The North Riding Sessions for 1608 refer to the sum of £3:6:8d, being for the repair of the causeway and pavement thereof. The year after, the North Riding was ordered to pay £27 for the repair of part of the bridge which was on the Yorkshire side, but nothing seems to have been done about it until July 1616, when a report was made that the bridge was still in a ruinous and decayed condition. Even then, nobody seemed to know who was responsible for dealing with the matter. Eventually, after many more reports of decay, including some in the very foundations of the piers, the Sessions at Thirsk on 8th April 1673 decided that the middle of the third pier adjoining the County of Durham should be the boundary between the two counties, and that the cost of repairs to that pier should be borne equally. Following this, an inscription as follows appeared on the parapet on the downstream side:

DUN.CONTRIBVAT NORTH RID.COM.EBOR.ET.COM
DUNEL.STATV. APVDSESS. VTRQ.GEN.PAC AN.DO 1673

thus marking the boundary between the two counties as being on the pier of the third arch from the Durham side. Some of the lettering is quite plain, but on the whole it is difficult to decipher today.

The bridge is a monumental affair, with seven arches, with ribbing on all but one. The arches are pointed, even on the upstream side where widening has taken place. The parapets rest on corbels which are decorated with carved heads on the downstream side. Alas, the features of the heads are very weather-worn.

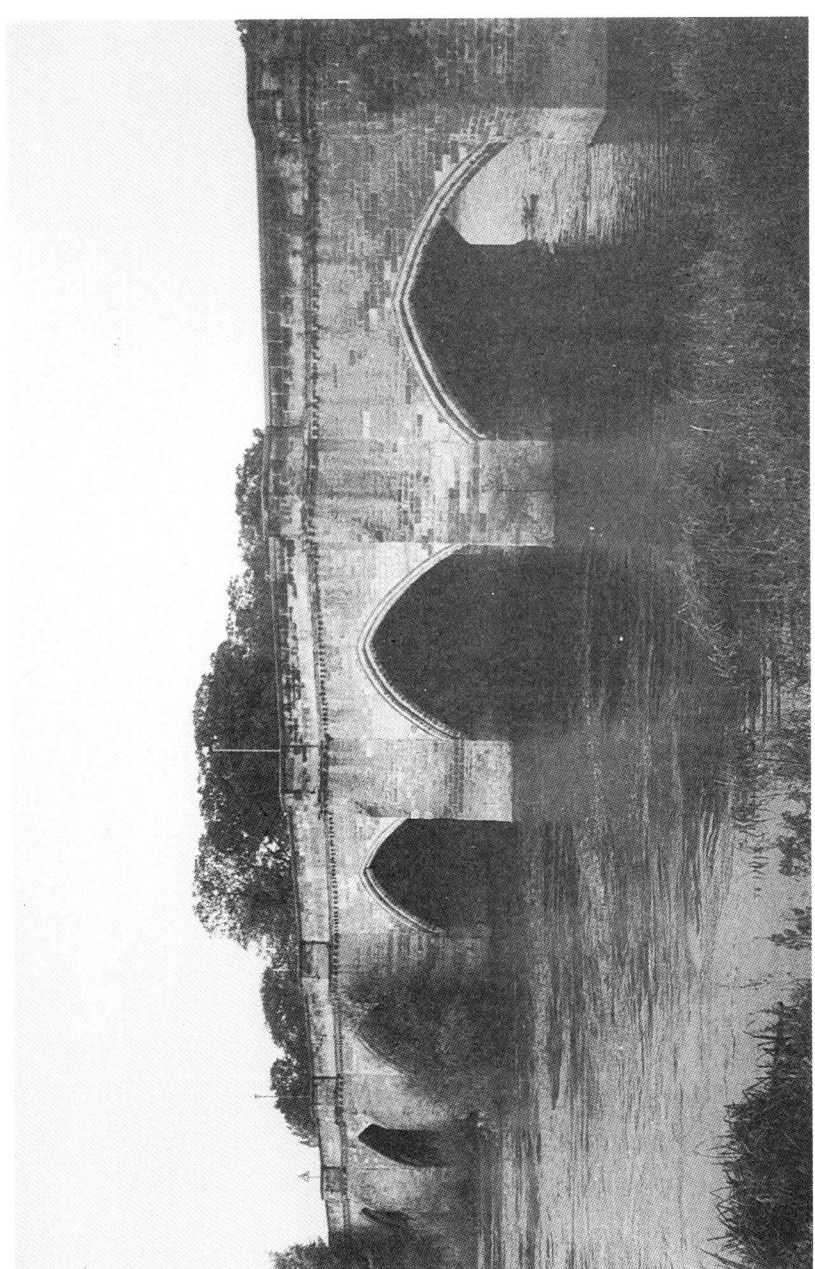

Croft Bridge

Croft Bridge withstood the great flood of February 1753, but the turnpike house suffered to the extent that the waters took it clean away, along with toll money. It is said that the flood at its height was over 15 ft above normal high water mark, and that the toll house was not the only building to suffer.

The high cutwaters allow for niches in the parapets (eight on each side) and the fascinating views of the river and its banks remain the same today as they did centuries ago, but on the Durham side the bank has been developed into pleasant parkland with seats. On the other side the church stands on high ground. The stonework of the bridge consists of not unattractive red and cream sandstone blocks in no special order, especially on the downstream side.

The church, rectory and the Croft Spa Hotel stand near this wonderful old bridge across the Tees. The hotel is a long Georgian affair with three-way pediment and porch. The church of St Peter's, like the bridge, is built of red and cream sandstone, and dates from the 14th century. Inside, the striking feature is the Millbanke two-bay pew which would have accommodated the whole family. It is reached by means of an oak staircase of 16 steps, and overlooks the congregation as well as the pulpit itself. The Millbanke tomb is there on the left of the nave, and on the other side is the tomb of Sir Richard Clervaux. If the church is locked, access can be gained by applying for the key at one of three sources, including the rectory and the hotel reception.

It is interesting to remember that Charles Dodgson, otherwise known as Lewis Carroll, the author of 'Alice in Wonderland', 'Through the Looking Glass' and many other writings from his vivid imagination, was the eldest son of the Rector of Croft, Archdeacon Dodgson. A plaque near the church door proclaims this. He went first to Richmond Grammar School, then to Rugby and Oxford. One can easily understand why he was, as a boy, intrigued with the curiously carved sedilia of three arches in the church; the bears, dragons and imps must have fired his imagination.

In 'The Two Brothers', another of Carroll's efforts, one brother hurls the other into the Tees at Croft Bridge:

> 'Thus shall he wallow about
>   And the fish take him at their ease
> For me to annoy it was ever his joy,
>   Now I'll teach him the meaning of "Tees!" ' '

Carroll seems to have been an artist, too, a caricaturist, perhaps: an illustration shows a school of fish, mouths agape ready to partake.

About that time, it is not difficult to imagine George Hudson, the railway king, leaning over the parapet of the bridge and pondering over the possibility of taking his railway from Croft over the Tees to join the famous 'Stockton and Darlington'.

Downstream, the Tees winds its way southwards and eastwards with very many loops. Eryholme, on the south bank on one of the loops, is an attractive village with a church of 11th century origin. There is also Neasham Hall. The river is full of interest here – it passes through red standstone cliffs and well-wooded country, comparatively quiet considering its proximity to Darlington. Then there is the old sulphur well with its traditional healing properties near Fishlock Weir.

Yet another surprising part of Old Yorkshire.

RIBBLESDALE

Among the many surprises in Upper Ribblesdale is Ling Gill.

At Ribblehead there is, of course, the famous railway viaduct now saved from almost certain closure, and an inn. Seen from here are Pen y Ghent, Whernside and Park Fell leading to Ingleborough, but hidden away in the bare hills to the north-east are three rivulets which feed the Ribble in no small measure. The most outstanding is Cam Beck, in the lower reaches of which is Ling Gill, a well-wooded ravine cutting deeply into the hillside. It is a nature reserve, but a genuine nature lover can gain access from Nether Lodge, a farmstead a mile or so down the valley of the Ribble, and reached on foot from Ingman Lodge just off the main road to Settle.

The gill, just short of half a mile long, is a naturalist's and geologist's paradise. There, among the flora and rocks, is an attractive waterfall. Towards the top end, enormous rocks have, through the ages, been split off the limestone cliffs, and strew the bottom in wild abandon. At the top of the ravine, just before the beck pours its copious waters into it, is the bridge. It is an ancient crossing, far from elegant but very attractive, and on the old packhorse way from Settle to Hawes, via Horton, High Birkwith, and Old Ing. One can hardly fail to notice a large stone set into the north parapet which proclaims:

AИИO   1765
THIS   BRIDGE
WAS   REPAIR
ED   AT   THE
CHARGE   OF
THE WHOLE W
EST   RIDEING

Repaired, the reader will note. It is said that it was built some 200 years before that.

Long gone are the packhorses, but now Pennine Way walkers tramp this route. Many halt awhile at this ancient spot and peer over, not without wonder, at the startlingly deep cleft into which the beck pours itself.

Following the track upstream for a short distance, one goes to the left and soon reaches the Roman road from Hawes to Ingleton. A bleaker spot, on all but a bright sunny day, is hard to imagine, but the panorama is memorable. Yet the Romans in their inimitable way drove their road over this high ground to reach their objectives. So where Roman soldiers once

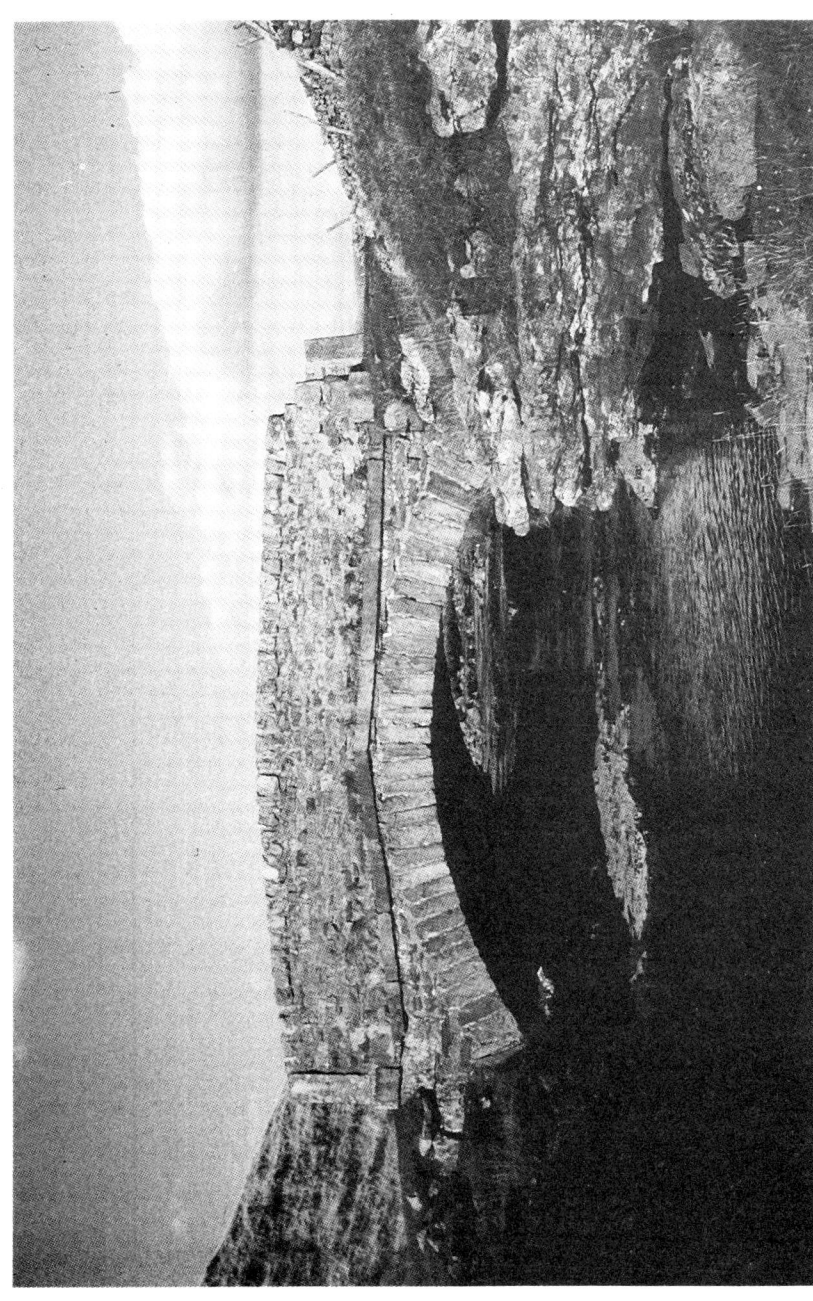

The bridge at Ling Gill

trod, perhaps not too enthusiastically, nearly two thousand years ago, we have 20th century walkers well past the halfway mark of the Pennine Way cheerfully making their way to the borders of Scotland, some 250 miles from the starting point at Edale in Derbyshire.

The second hidden valley is that of the Gayle Beck. At Thorn's Gill, the water cuts through a miniature limestone gorge which can be reached quite easily from the main Ribblehead – Hawes road just before the former Gearstones Inn. The field path leads one to a wee packhorse bridge without parapets. The bridge crosses the actual ravine and is, therefore, unlike Ling Gill, high above the water. At first sight the bridge looks a flimsy affair, and for some years iron stays have kept the stonework in position. Now that repairs have been made it gives one more confidence than hitherto. Here again, as in the case of Ling Gill, the flora and indeed the bird life add to its attractiveness in this hidden valley cut in limestone. Hereabouts are enormous blocks of limestone, not in the ravine itself, but scattered around on the greensward adjacent to the path on the eastern side of the beck. They have been around from time immemorial – maybe the ice age. The gill is about half a mile in length, and at the head is a wooden bridge from which there is a magnificent view of Ingleborough and Whernside.

God's Bridge is our third attraction. To reach this, and incidentally cross Brow Gill beck, the finger-post at Nether Lodge directing one to High Birkwith should be followed up the hill. Suddenly Brow Gill appears. There is nothing very spectacular here, except that the bridge is as God made it. The track, quite wide, passes over the water by means of a grass-grown limestone bridge with man-made stone walls as 'parapets'. Over the bridge, the track from High Birkwith to Old Ing is reached, and with it once more the Pennine Way. High Birkwith is an ancient place and once belonged to Jervaulx Abbey. In packhorse days it was a flourishing wayside inn.

At the head of the Brow Gill is an interesting cave of easy access from which the beck issues. The water can be followed underground as far as Calf Holes where the beck is swallowed adjacent to the Pennine Way leading to Ling Gill. This little adventure is not suitable for the inexperienced.

STAINFORTH

The next bridge of special note is at Stainforth, some miles down the Ribble Valley. The long straight road from High Birkwith is metalled and undulates somewhat, until it enters Horton-in-Ribblesdale, where two modest bridges almost meet at the Crown Inn, where the main road crosses, the Ribble, and then over Brants Gill. Lower down still, and just before reaching Stainforth village, one turns down a steep and narrow lane to a gem of Ribblesdale.

At Stainforth, the Ribble forsakes the village and glides down the bottom of a steep-sided valley a few hundred yards to the west, leaving the Cowside Beck and its stepping stones to add to the charm of the village. The beck joins the Ribble where the valley widens out a little, and where the discretely hidden railway disappears under the old mansion of Taitlands.

Meanwhile, the Ribble passes under a masterpiece of a packhorse bridge, and within a hundred yards or so cascades down a series of limestone ledges, finally falling in one great plunge into a deep pool. Stainforth Foss is an attractive waterfall and, with its wooded background and easy approach, set in such picturesque surroundings, must surely rank as one of the loveliest sections of the whole of the Ribble's course, thanks in no small measure to the Craven Fault, the famous upthrust of rock which occurred many eons ago.

But the jewel in the crown must surely be the packhorse bridge itself. A 17th century affair, but obviously repaired since that time, it has, like so many other packhorse bridges, one graceful (almost semi-circular) arch. Instead of a long approach at each end, Stainforth has but one; the east end comes to an abrupt finish due to a steep lane leading down to it from the by-pass road. The bridge is a little wider than most of its kind, but only wide enough to allow small vehicles to pass over it. The view of its from almost any direction makes a delightful picture. It is cared for by the National Trust, and so we can be assured that it will give pleasure to future generations.

The long approach to the bridge, though steep, starts at the hamlet of Knight Stainforth. It is thought that one Samuel Watson, who built Knight Stainforth Hall c. 1670, also saw to the building of the bridge, which would connect Clapham with Malham. Watson was an ardent Quaker and suffered assault and persecution. The Hall has a venerable and ancient appearance. Note the blocked-up windows of the top floor – presumably blocked up to avoid at least some of the inequitous window tax. Other windows may well have been opened since those days.

An ancient well exists at the road junction above the Hall, but it does not seem to be very active at the time of writing.

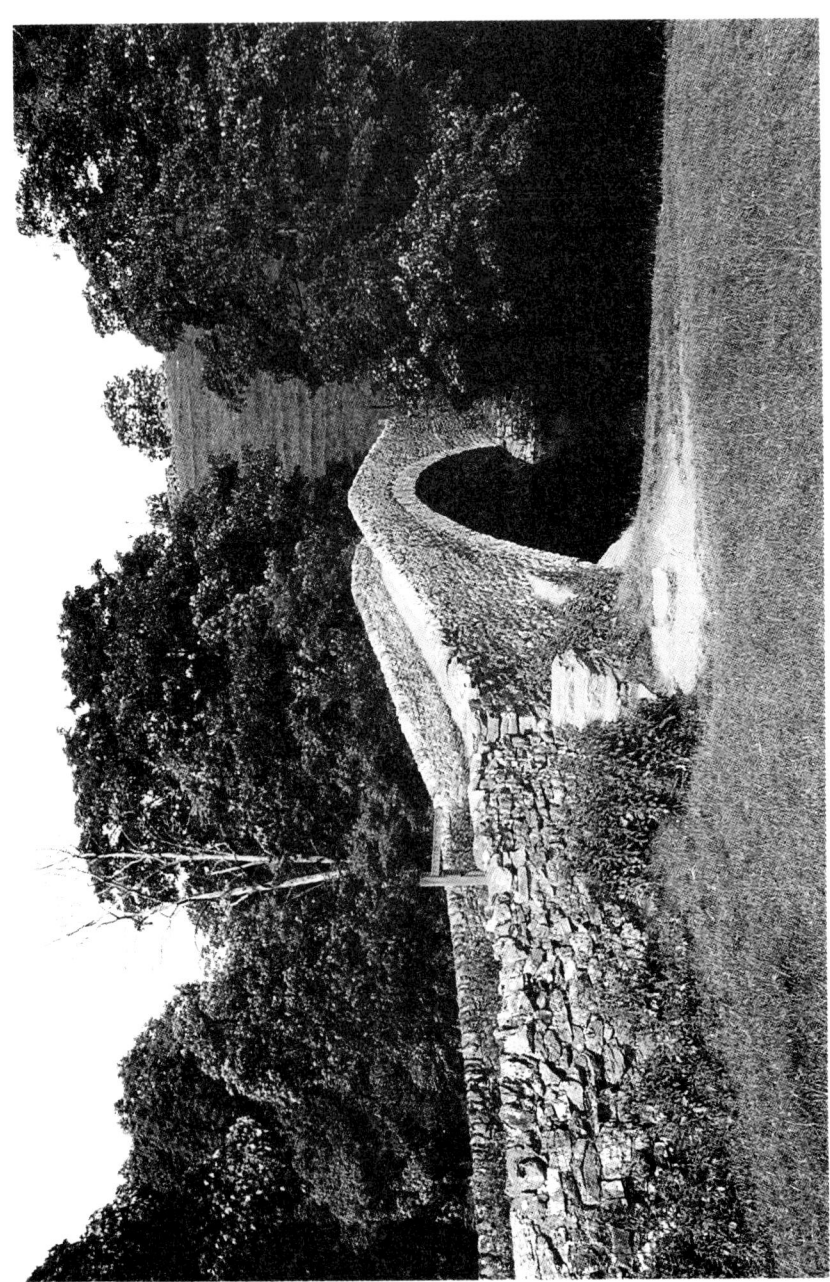

Stainforth packhorse bridge

The Ribble is well worth following downstream until it is joined by the Hodder, which forms part of the old Yorkshire boundary near Great Mytton, the latter still being in the Yorkshire diocese of Bradford.

On the way to Great Mytton, we pass over Settle Bridge. Originally, this was a narrow structure and was widened in 1837, and, until the Settle bypass was constructed during the past decade, carried an enormous amount of traffic, heavy and light. The oldest part of the bridge is on the north side.

At Long Preston, we turn right and, soon after passing over the railway, we reach Cow Bridge on the way to Wigglesworth. It is well worthy of note for it has no less than seven arches, but the river passes under only one, a wide segmented structure. The smaller arches at each end enable a long approach to be made, and obviate the need for a hump in the middle. The river glides quietly along through pastoral country up and down stream, though to prevent flooding, the banks are built up.

The next crossing of note is at Paythorne. Here the Ribble passes through a defile, but immediately past the bridge it enters pastoral country again. The bridge has three pointed arches which suggest great age, and at each end the approach from north and south comes down the side of the valley obliquely. It will be seen that on the north-east end the stonework has been built up subsequent to the original building, making a long approach to the river. On the south-east end on the upstream side is a track leading upwards, from which an attractive picture can be painted or photographed.

From Gisburn, a series of bridges across the Ribble leads us to Great Mitton. On the way is Sawley, with its abbey, and the famous archway, which now stands at the side of the road hard by the Spread Eagle Inn. Around Great Mitton are three bridges. Before reaching Great Mitton is the famous Eadsford Bridge with its ancient pointed arches. On the bridge itself the words LCC EADSFORD BRIDGE are carved on one parapet, which reminds us we must surely be in Lancashire! The road from Clitheroe descends steeply to the bridge, and on the other side the road ascends just as steeply to the Edisford Inn, with its sign depicting the bridge with rounded arches, obviously painted from the downstream side, which has been widened. Now we are in an area which was formerly Yorkshire, but still in the diocese of Bradford (West Yorkshire). There is Little Mytton Hall, a Tudor residence, and in Great Mitton itself is a pearl of a church, high up from the Ribble, rich in monumental work, for example the Sherburn Chapel commemorating Sir Richard Sherburn who founded Stonyhurst. The Ribble is crossed here by Mytton Bridge, the last of our Yorkshire bridges over that river. Here we must cross into Lancashire, first by the

Higher Hodder Bridge, with the dividing line between the two counties duly marked on the parapet. The Lower Hodder Bridge is our objective, because a short distance before the Hodder joins the Ribble is the unusual sight of a three-arched packhorse bridge, a full view of which is gained from the modern bridge. The arches are segmental; the middle one is of great span and rises to a considerable height, the other two being of different size but still large. Giant cutwaters divide the three. The river is very wide here, and appears to have been fordable at one time in the distant past. There are no approach roads apparent at the present time, and at one end fencing bars one from an attempt at crossing the bridge, a wise precaution. At the other end, approach is difficult and there are no parapets, though large stones hereabouts suggest their existence at one time.

The bridge is known as Cromwell's Bridge because Cromwell, on his march from Gisburn to Preston, crossed the Hodder at this point, presumably over the bridge, in 1648. On the evening of the 16th August of that year he quartered his army in the field adjoining Stonyhurst Hall, he himself spending the night in the hall. Seeing that his host was a Royalist as well as a papist, he dreaded assassination, and is said to have had a large table placed in the dining hall upon which he spent the night, his pistols and sword at his side!

It is said that Sir Richard Sherburn built the bridge in 1561, to replace a much earlier one.

DENTDALE

On our travels between the head of Ribblesdale and the head of Wensleydale, we are usually in a hurry, but it is good to take a break and drop down into Dentdale and have a quick look at the bridges in this far-flung outpost of the Diocese of Bradford.

The dale is unique, differing in so many ways from its counterparts in the south and east. A quainter place than Dent town itself would be hard to find. Apart from this, and its little close neighbour, Gawthrop, the whole valley has no villages as such and consists mainly of farmsteads scattered at intervals along the sides of the hills, especially Rise Hill, which comes down in great sweeps to the river Dee. There is, of course, the hamlet of Lea Yeat some four miles up river from Dent, but it is just a hamlet.

From its beginning, the river Dee tumbles down a series of slabs of limestone. From Lea Yeat onwards, the water calms down, and, although passing over limestone beds for the most part, continues on its quiet way down the valley. There are one or two exceptions, such as Hud's Foss, but let us stop at Lea Yeat for a moment or two where there are three bonny one-arched stone bridges within a few hundred yards of each other. The first is at Lea Yeat itself. It is narrow, but wide enough for most modestly-sized vehicles. It has seen drovers, packhorses and coal carts as well as tumbrels (unusual wooden carts with two wheels integral with the axle – especially well-known in old Dentdale). The bridge is a comely affair and forms a lovely picture with the dwellings and trees nearby; it is somewhat larger than the other two. The next bridge is reached by means of a riverside path (part of the modern Dalesway) only a few hundred yards in length. It is called Ewegales Bridge, and is well-maintained with a shallow arch spanning the Dee. We cross this and take the road to the right to Cowgill, where there is yet another crossing – this time over Cowgill Beck. This is really an ancient bridge, and although there is ample evidence of new cement pointing, there is a stone slab which bears the following legend:

THIS
BRIDG REPER
ED AT THE
CHARG OF TH
WEST RIDING
A.D.1702

The letter E has been omitted from the words 'bridge', the final 'the', and 'charge', it will be noted. The spelling of 'repaired' will also be noted.

The ends of the bridge almost seem to have become part of the living rock on which they are based, and nothing short of an earthquake or an inter-continental lorry would be capable of breaking them down. It is thought by many to be the gem of crossings, perhaps with one exception, in the whole of Dentdale. Nearby is the little church of St John, built on the site of a former Presbyterian chapel. We turn east over the bridge and soon reach Lea Yeat again, wondering why the road from there did not follow the course of the present footpath to Ewegales Bridge, which would serve Cowgill as well as the two roads down the Dale.

Downstream at Dent town, there is the Church Bridge, a more modern affair than the three we have just left, but nonetheless attractive and replacing an ancient crossing.

The Craven Old Way, an old packhorse route from Dent to Ingleton, goes up the dale to Deepdale Foot and over the shoulder of Whernside. A drover's road followed this route part way, and joined the Turbary Road on the slopes of Leck Fell on its way to Kirkby Lonsdale. The drovers also used the road from Kirkby Stephen via Garsdale Head to Dent. The old Coal Road went this way, as coal was mined between Dent Railway Station and Garsdale Head.

So while Dent would not witness a great deal of the romance of the old coaching days, as did the Great North Road and the old A6 through Kendal, it had its moments.

As we leave Dent town, the scenery gradually changes. The river ceases to flow over limestone slabs and pebbles are seen at its bed. Before the Dee joins the Rathay approaching Sedbergh, there are two other bridges well worth noting. The first is Barth Bridge, and the second is Rash Bridge, a beautiful, very high arched stone structure in well-wooded surroundings. Small corbels appear to give partial support to the parapets. Unlike so many of the bridges in Upper Dentdale, its arch is almost semicircular, and the waters do not seem to be in such a hurry in normal weather conditions. In fact, one should not fail to linger here – there is much bird life, and fish abound at certain times in one particular deep pool. Artists and photographers, too, find a scramble down the river bank quite rewarding.

WENSLEYDALE AND ITS BRIDGES

The river Ouse, or the Ure as it is called in its upper and middle reaches, rises on the old border of Westmorland.

Thwaite Bridge, which carries the Sedbergh-Hawes road, first recorded in 1775, is now relatively modern. Near Bainbridge the Ure received two tributaries: the Bain, the outflow of Semerwater, and Sargill Beck, which drains the slopes of Abbotside and is finally known as Grange Gill. The latter pours its water over the lip of a limestone cove – a miniature Hardraw Scar – and under an ancient packhorse bridge, Bow Bridge, which carried the old road to Sedbergh. The Sedbergh road now ignores the loop to the north, and crosses the Gill at its deepest point via the Bainbridge road.

Bow Bridge is attributed to the monks of the short-lived Fors Abbey and so dates back to the 12th century. At present it has no parapets. The arch is semicircular, and underneath the ribbing can plainly be seen. However, in the 18th century it was widened to twice its original width, but without ribbing. The whole is now grass-grown and can easily be missed by the average traveller, as it lies to the north of the modern road and half-hidden by houses, comprising what is left of the hamlet which once stood around it. Some of the buildings disappeared when the modern road was widened. Bow Bridge can be seen by entering a paddock through a gate on the left of the lane leading northward. It is interesting to note that this lane meets up with Lady Ann Clifford's road down the valley, and, while standing on this ancient crossing at Bow Bridge and resting awhile, one's mind can picture pack-horses and colourful stagecoaches passing this way.

Curiously enough, Fors Abbey, or the very scant remains of it, lies further down the valley of Grange Gill, and a track to it starts near the modern bridge. Following this track, we come to Hockett Bridge across the Gill. It is little more than a footbridge and its history is hard to come by. However, it was described by Edmund Bogg over a hundred years ago as 'an ancient, quaint, grey, narrow one-arched packhorse bridge under which splashes Grange Beck, at any time forming a charming picture'. It still does. Furthermore cattle come to drink there. They stand in the water and appear to meditate. Passing through the former supports of the railway track a little downstream, we come to a footbridge across the water and reach a substantial farmhouse. A number of stones used to build the house are obviously from the Abbey of Fors which is reputed to have stood here. From the footpath between the railway embankment and the house, one obtains a view of a trefoil-headed window built into the stonework of the back of the house wall, an obvious remnant of the one-time Abbey which,

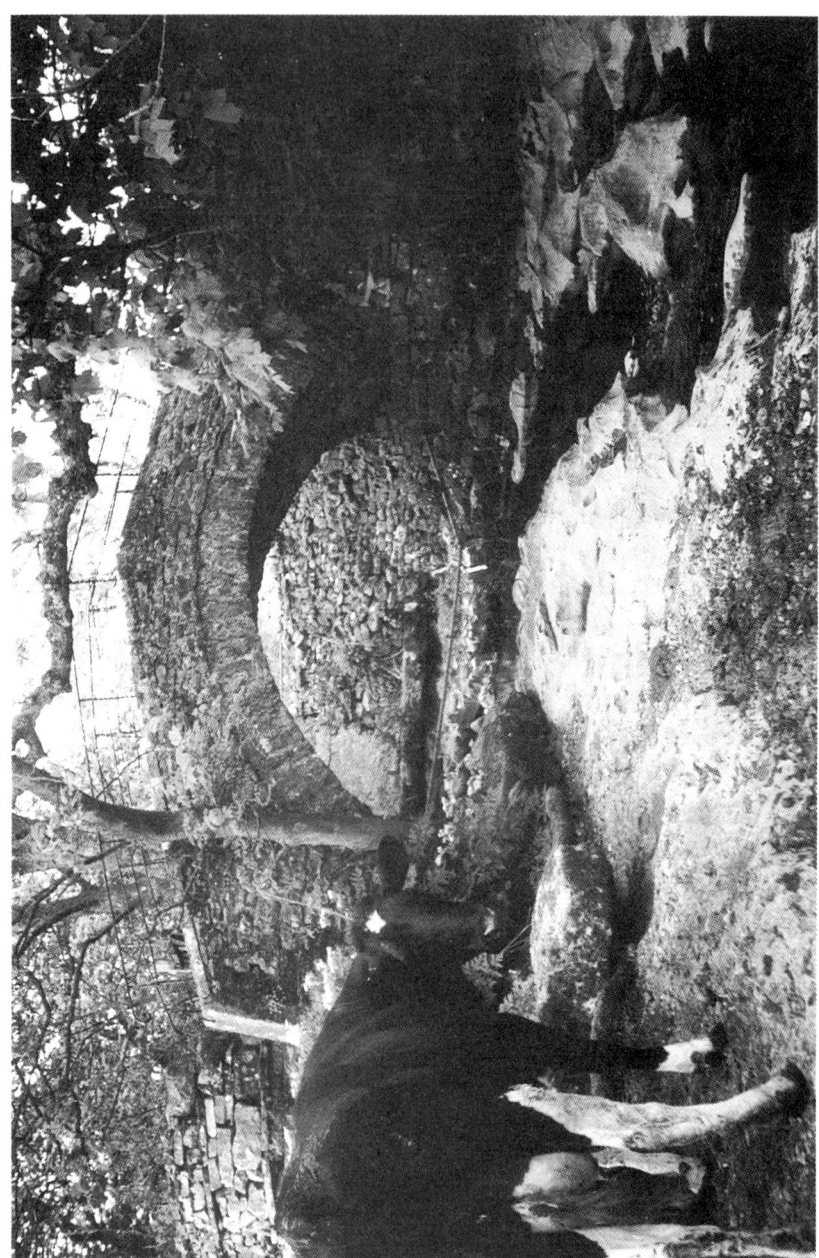

Hockett Bridge, near Askrigg

after only 11 years, moved to Jervaulx at the eastern end of Wensleydale.

An alternative and pleasant approach to the little old bridge and the site of Fors Abbey is from the north end of Yore Bridge, over which the road from Bainbridge reaches Askrigg. Yore Bridge has three segmental arches and may date from the 18th century. In July 1607, the then bridge, like so many others, was stated to be 'in great ruin and decaie'. Following that, the sum of £20 was levied for its repair. The flagged path from Yore Bridge through the fields leaves the river and veers towards Askrigg and the former railway, the farm at Fors, and, of course, the wee bridge. If one carries on past the farmhouse, one eventually reaches Askrigg by crossing the old railway track. In 1877, the railway invaded the upper dale and, like so many country stations, kept a respectful distance from the village or township – even so, it put Askrigg on the map again, especially the tourist map. What a wonderful opening-up of the valley for the Victorian and Edwardian tourist; everything untouched by modern 'progress'. Then came the motor, and more and more motor vehicles providing door-to-door transport. The year 1954 saw the end of the railway. A little further along the road towards Askrigg from where the railway station stood is another flagged path through the fields which leads one to the churchyard and the Market Square in which stood the lovely Old Hall, one of the outstanding buildings in Wensleydale generally and in Askrigg in particular. The author was fortunate in taking a photograph of it before it suffered the fatal fire in 1935.

Askrigg is more or less its own parish, but was formerly included in the hugh parish of Aysgarth, the largest in Yorkshire. Once a village, Askrigg became a town, and is now once again a village. When it was a town, one would have found a cotton mill, clockmakers, forges, dyehouses, more than one grocer, saddlers, knitters and weavers and so on, and, up in the hills, lead mining. Even though Askrigg received its market charter as late as 1587, and Hawes did not receive its charter until 1700, eventually Hawes outstripped Askrigg in importance and, of course, along with Leyburn has been a market town of importance for very many years. Askrigg once saw a stream of pack-horses and had no less than five inns. Then came the turnpike roads: Richmond to Lancaster via Askrigg to Sedbergh. Later came the railway, and now motor cars and lorries!

AYSGARTH

Aysgarth is, of course, famous for its falls, which occur at just about the narrowest part of the Wensleydale valley. How frequently do we admire the bridge itself? We lean over its parapet and admire the Upper Falls and then walk downstream and admire the Middle and Lower Falls, taking the old one-arched bridge for granted.

Originally, it was a packhorse structure nine feet wide. It was built in 1594 with money left by a Sedbergh gentleman, James Sedgwick. The money was stated to amount to £6:13:4d, but by 1637 it was reported that it was in ruins. No wonder, one may believe. However, a substantial stone bridge with a single semi-circular arch stands astride the Ure as it has done for many years now. It has a span of 20 yards. The Ure pursues a fairly tranquil course, but at Aysgarth its character changes, not once but three times in a comparatively short space. The Upper Falls are wide and fill the suddenly narrowing valley, and by the time the water reaches the bridge the valley has become V-shaped. The approaches by road on the village side are very steep, and on the north side the land is so steep that the approach takes a devious route before turning sharply left to make the crossing. Just before leaving the bridge, we note that it was widened considerably on the downstream side, as can be seen by the somewhat different character of the stonework. A little downstream, then, are the Middle Falls, and a path through countless hazel bushes leads one to the Lower Falls, thought by some to be the most spectacular. Further downstream the river loses its tranquillity until it reaches Redmire's more gentle falls. Thereafter the water flows quietly along.

Curiously enough, the large new car park and information centre are on the opposite side of the valley from the village, in much the same way that the old railway station was in relation to the village. Halfway up the hill to the village is the church, whose parish dominated much of the dale. Little is left of the original 12th century building, the base of the tower and two piscinae being still in evidence. At the top of the hill there used to be a hospice for palmers, or pilgrims. The site is now a hotel, The Palmer Flatts. The village itself consists mainly of a long main street, on the top side of which there is a plaque to the memory of the late Dr William Pickles (1885–1968), one of the best known and lovable general practitioners of all time. A great epidemiologist, born in Leeds, he practised in Aysgarth, and travelled the world in the course of his work into the bargain.

The number of times he crossed Aysgarth Bridge in the course of his merciful missions, day and night, will never be known.

WENSLEY

Wensley received its Charter for a market as long ago as 1202, and it was renewed in 1306/7 by James de Wendeslaye, at which time a weekly market on Mondays and a yearly fair were held. Struck by the Black Death in 1563 more badly than many places, Wensley relapsed into a small village and its market gave way to Askrigg, and later to Leyburn and Hawes. Nevertheless, Wensley parish includes Leyburn, and what a lovely church of Holy Trinity stands there, clothed with its light grey sundrenched stones. It houses a magnificent collection of antiquities, and should not be missed.

Roads from several directions meet at Wensley, which lacks the hardness of many Dales villages. The main road from Leyburn to Hawes crosses the Ure by Wensley Bridge. So many visitors to the Dales cross the river at this point, yet are quite unaware of this historic bridge, perhaps because it lacks a hump in the middle.

According to Dorothy Wordsworth, sister of the famous William, her brother took his bride from Brompton near Scarborough to Grasmere, via Wensley Bridge and West Witton ('the long village along the side of a hill'). Even a cursory look at the bridge inspires a close inspection. One finds that, like so many other ancient crossings, it has been widened on one side only. Viewed from upstream, there are four rounded arches, three of which are almost the same size. However, the fourth supports the northern end and is only half-size. The huge and well-cut stones used give an impressive, if somewhat stark, appearance, but the pointed cutwaters, of a stepped variety, look as if they are much older than the arches and parapet. The widening and restoration took place in 1818. The view of the bridge from downstream is a delightful one. Two pointed arches of ancient stone allow the passage of the main stream, whilst a large rounded one at the south end and a small one at the north end complete the picture. It is not surprising that artists and photographers are attracted to the riverbank downstream where a public footpath continues from upstream. The tree trunks at the water's edge on the opposite side are beautifully reflected in the river at normal level.

According to Leland the 'great Bridge of stone was made many yere sins by a good Person of Wencelaw caullid Alwine'. Richard, Lord Scrope of Bolton, in his will, made the year 1400, left £40 for the repair of Wensley Bridge. In 1587 the repairs cost £60. Alwine died in 1430.

It would appear that the large rounded arch replacing a pointed one enabled the carriageway to be levelled out, and possibly the little arch did the same.

Crossing the bridge from south to north, one immediately senses something different about Wensley village. Its tiny Post Office on the right of the sloping green belongs to another age. In spite of the lack of the great elm tree which once graced the green, it still has a gracious appearance. The elm, by the by, was destroyed in 1946 as a result of the great gale that year. The old-world character is enhanced by the grand entrance gates of Bolton Hall, and on the left of the gates is the entrance to the Dower House. Bolton Hall is, of course, the seat of Lord Bolton, through the daughter of the last of the Scrope family of Castle Bolton fame.

Upstream is another lovely old bridge. It crosses the Ure and leads directly from the main road to Bolton Hall itself. It has two segmental arches and pointed cutwaters which rise to the top of the parapets with niches. At the north end of each parapet is a tall square column surmounted by a stone ball, giving the whole structure some dignity. On the downstream side, carved in the stonework, is the inscription:

C D B
1733

suggesting the date it was built or rebuilt.

The bridge is unfit for motors, and a warning notice to this effect appears near the Lodge, where the lane leaves the main road and leads to this gracious crossing.

COVERDALE

Let us now retrace our steps and explore Coverdale. The Cover valley winds its way westward from Cover Bridge, and a delightful way to reach it is by way of a very minor road from East Witton village, passing Braithwaite Hall (National Trust) on one's left. The road then leads directly to Coverham Abbey Bridge. This is a very ancient bridge with a single span of about 17 yards, wide enough for most vehicles. Leland refers to it as being a 'very little above this Priorye', but for once it does not seem to have been in a ruinous state! The pointed arch has double arch rings, built in one plane, and springs from chamfered entablatures. At low water one can pass under the bridge, on the stonework, onto a pebble beach downstream. Leland had been in other realms for some 65 years before it is recorded that the bridge was in a state of great decay (1615 Sessions), and the sum of £30 was spent on repairs during the ensuing 45 years. The area is a fascinating one. First we have Coverham Abbey, most of the ruins of which stand in the garden of a house largely built of abbey stones. The approach is along a short lane and under an ancient archway. It is not normally open to visitors, but the arches of an arcade (the chief remains) can be plainly seen at fairly close quarters from the lane. Curiously carved stones abound.

At the end of the little road from East Witton, and on the south end of Coverham Abbey Bridge, the road rises towards Caldbergh Bridge. This is a comparatively modern bridge and the average motorist would hardly notice that it crosses a limestone gorge of surprising depth. Its parapets are like a neatly-built field wall with the usual capping, but not the dry-stone variety. The road surface shows not the slightest rise towards the middle. On one side, carved in a smooth slab set into the wall, are the words 'CALD-BERGH BRIDGE' and on the opposite side is the caption in stone 'NYR 1933'. If you raise your head after reading the latter, you gaze down a tree-clothed gorge. The scene following a quick thaw of snow on the hills is awesome. Just a very short distance upstream is an ancient packhorse bridge, grass-grown and without parapets. It is Ulla Bridge, which crosses the limestone gorge near the top. This packhorse bridge consists of three very narrow arches side by side, duly integrated into a single one of comparatively good width. Naturally, it was built at the narrowest and shallowest part of the gorge. The old market road from the Leyburn area to Kettlewell would presumably go via Carlton on the other side of the valley, but maybe Ulla Bridge would be used on the one-time route to the head of Nidderdale, via West Scrafton on the south side of the Cover valley.

A little way up the road from Caldbergh Bridge is a field path on the left,

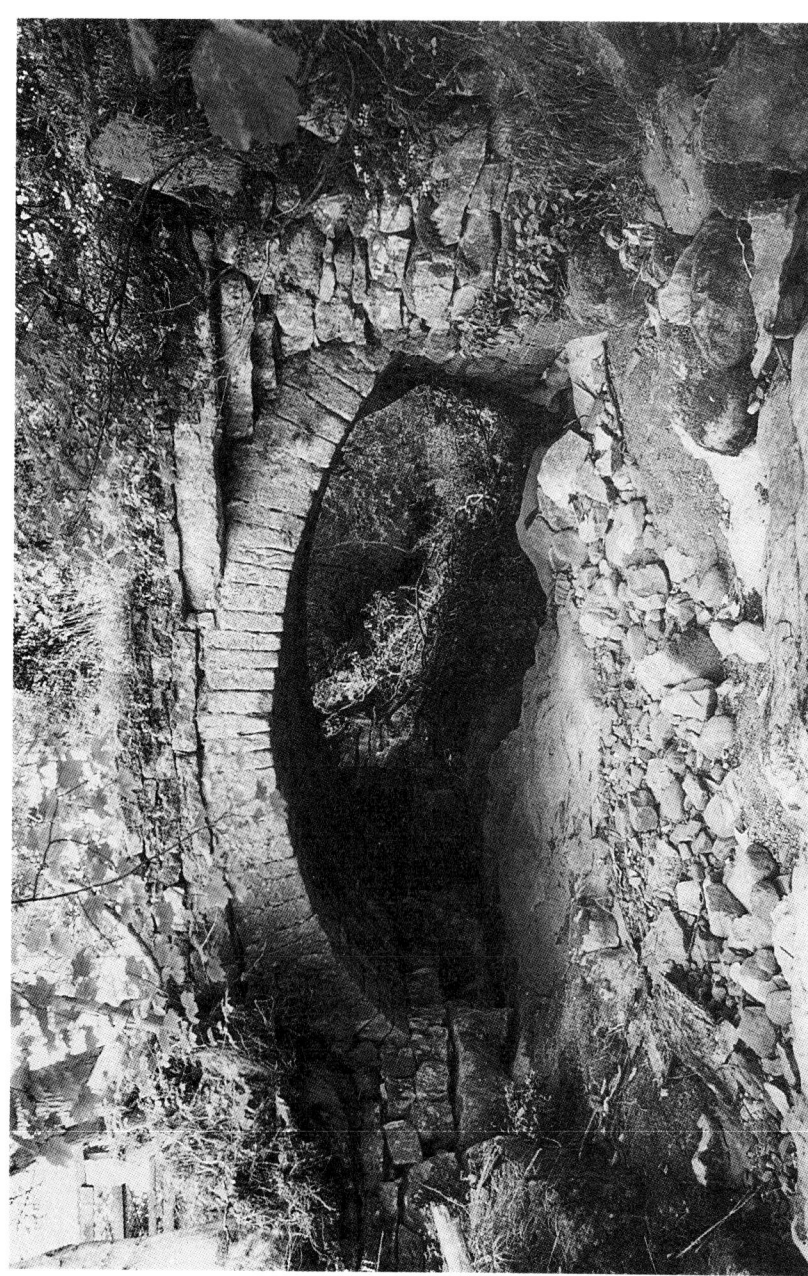

Ulla Bridge

taking one to a series of stone steps leading obliquely down the steep-sided valley to St Simon's Chapel near the river. No archway or remains of windows can be seen, just stone walls of no great height. Two enormous trees have taken root within the grass-grown walls. The chapel was built some 600 years ago, and a hermit, who lived in part of it, kept it in order under the watchful eyes of the monks of Coverham Abbey until the Dissolution, sometime after which it is said to have been an ale-house for a space. Upstream from the remains of St Simon's Chapel is a footpath which leads to St Simon's Bridge, a very modern timber affair, and indeed very substantial. It spans a wide part of the river and is based on large stone abutments which seem to have been built on much older foundations. Across this bridge is a pleasant footpath leading to Melmerby village on the north side of the valley.

THE WONDERFUL TRIO

Cover Bridge, Ulshaw and Kilgram – of the three, little one-arched Cover Bridge must surely carry far more traffic than the other two put together. It is, of course, on the main route up and down the Wensleydale valley from Jervaulx Abbey to Hawes and beyond.

East Witton village, thought by many to be the gem of Wensleydale, is almost by-passed by the main road. As soon as it enters the village it turns sharply north, so the cottages on each side of the extensive green are spared the ceaseless passing of traffic. The village is said to have been planned by the monks of Jervaulx in early medieval times. However, the main road must be followed to reach Cover Bridge, the last one over the Cover before it sidles quietly into the Ure almost unnoticed. One cannot refer to Cover Bridge without mentioning its ancient hostelry, the Cover Bridge Inn. Prior to World War II, the Inn had been kept by the Towler family, who were in possession of the recipe for Wensleydale cheese used by the monks of Jervaulx at the time of the Dissolution. For fishing or walking, along the riversides or the hills and visiting castles and abbeys, the area can have few equals as a centre. The bridge can be viewed easily from up or down stream and consists of one almost semi-circular arch, but each parapet appears to rise to a point at the centre forming a very obtuse angle. It consists of double arch rings, built in two orders, a truly remarkable bridge in that it supports all manner of traffic day in and day out, week in and week out. An earlier-known bridge, which is said to have existed here in medieval times, was destroyed in 1608, and rebuilt in 1673 at a cost of £85. The present bridge is an 18th century affair.

Instead of taking the main road to Leyburn and Middleham, we take the road straight ahead after crossing Cover Bridge, and a few hundred yards leads us to Ulshaw Bridge which crosses the Ure. Compared with little Cover Bridge, Ulshaw is a massive affair, yet it is only 12 feet from parapet to parapet. The six massive cutwaters allow for recesses for foot passengers – very necessary in such a narrow bridge. In a recess on the upstream side is a sundial on a pedestal, which is inscribed 'R W 1674' and has a list to starboard. There are four segmental arches which carry 22 yards of carriageway. Downstream, the banks of the river are well-wooded, but upstream the views are of open country. Once again, we cannot ignore the reports of John Leland, who from 1533 to 1539 travelled the country on a commission from Henry VIII. He does not actually refer specifically to Ulshaw (or Ullsey) Bridge, but he certainly crossed the river by a ford when approaching Middleham from the north. On another occasion he said that the bridge over the Ure by Middleham was of timber, but a stone bridge seems to have existed in 1588 when much repair work was done. Whilst on the subject of repairs, it is quite remarkable that as much as £1000 is said to have been spent on it.

Going back to the 7th century, the story goes that at this crossing of the Ure, St Oswin, King of Deira, a devout Christian, dispersed his army (rather than have bloodshed over the dispute with King Oswei regarding boundaries) and retired to Gilling where he was slain on the command of the King of Bernicia. The latter later repented, and built and endowed a monastery as reparation for his sins. Curiously enough, just north of the bridge is a Roman Catholic establishment at the present time.

It is also interesting to note that it was here that East Witton market was held, as a temporary measure, during the plague of 1563, but it never returned to the village. There is a choice of routes here across the bridge. Kilgram Bridge being our objective, we take the road eastward which more or less follows the river, but deviates a little leaving Danby and Thornton Steward between us and the water. Soon after leaving the road to Thornton Steward, we turn quite suddenly to the right and find ourselves on Kilgram Bridge.

Kilgram is best seen in the morning sunshine on the downstream side. Said to have been built by the Normans, and associated with the monks of Jervaulx (12th century), subsequent floods swept it and its successors into the turbulent waters of the Ure. We know that it was in good repair as long ago as 1585.

The name Kilgram seems to have been the result of a story of the Devil himself, who offered to rebuild the bridge on condition that the first living creature to cross it after completion should be sacrificed to him. A shepherd swam across the river first, and then called for his dog called Grim, who crossed the bridge to meet his master at the other side. When the dog was about to run up to his master, it suddenly collapsed and died. What a pity the shepherd didn't arrange for a lamb to cross the bridge instead of his faithful dog. A sacrificial lamb!

There is another story – the bridge is supposed to be one stone short, so that it would never be finished and so defeat Satan's condition. If that stone were inserted, then Heaven help those who crossed the bridge after the insertion of that fateful stone. The whereabouts of the gap in which the missing stone might have been placed has eluded the author.

And so the grand old bridge of six segmental arches of stone slumbers on. As one stands on that narrow bridge, looking upstream or down, the hurly-burly of modern traffic is forgotten. Serenity is the order of the day.

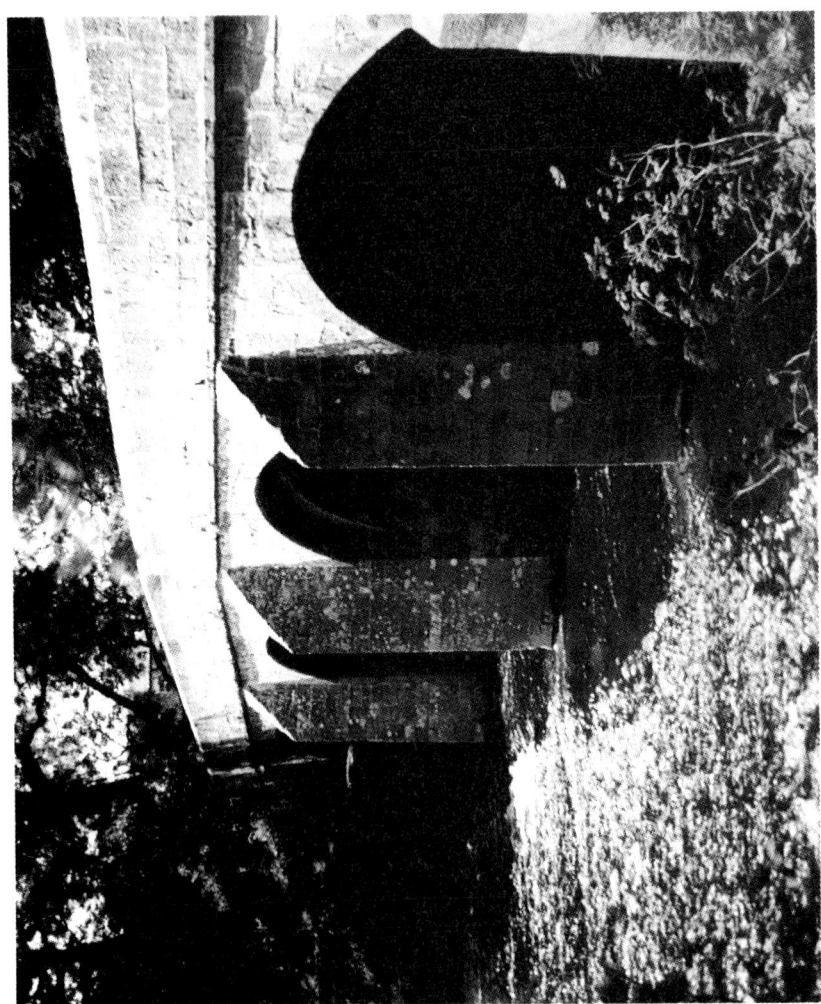

Kilgram Bridge

In the spring and early summer, birds sing their songs without being disturbed, and the wild flowers bloom once again. After flowing smoothly over the paved riverbed under the arches, the waters splash over the edge to their natural bed, on their way to the next crossing at Masham some eight miles to the east.

At the east side of the approach road from the north is a stone arched footway, just before it reaches the bridge, a thoughtful adjunct to avoid flood waters across a pronounced dip in the road.

Going downstream to Masham, Jervaulx Abbey must not be missed. Whilst suffering by comparison only with Fountains, Jervalux has plenty of charm. Here are the remains of the once-great abbey only some 10 miles away from the site at Fors, near Askrigg, from which the holy men moved after a very short time.

Jervaulx has a character of its own, and somehow one feels one is standing on very sacred ground. There are no crowds of visitors, no huge car parks, no official guides and cafes, which surely contribute to this feeling. There is a hush about the place, which adds to the serenity which so long ago descended upon it. Before the Dissolution, there would, of course, have been much activity apart from the devotional side of life – the sale of wool, for example.

I suppose one should recommend a visit towards the end of a summer evening, as the sun goes down and the first stars begin to show. A song thrush perched high above ground, almost bursting its little throat with lovely notes, would, for most mortals, help to create 'atmosphere'. Time for Vespers and Compline.

MASHAM AND SWINTON

Masham – the hollow in the hills where Mass was held, or so it is said.

How far does its history go? Possibly the Bronze Age, c.1500 BC. Then came the Romans, in the first century, and occupied Masahamshire for 300 years; the Danes and Saxons followed and then the Normans. The church at Masham was referred to in the Domesday Book and a great deal of the town's history revolves round the church. A Saxon Cross in the churchyard is a unique survival of the 9th century. It is a massive affair of several tiers, with figures carved in the arcades. The church tower has a full peal of bells and the following epitaph is worth noting:

> Here lies an old ringer, beneath the cold clay
> Who has rung many peals both to serious and gay;
> Thro' grandsires triplets with ease he could range
> Till death called his Bob and brought round his last change.

The market place consists of a huge square with a cross mounted on steps with trees all around. The town was originally granted a Charter in AD 1250 to hold a market on Fridays, and a second charter was granted in the 14th century. A two-day sheep fair is held on the Assumption of the Virgin in September as well as a modest weekly market on Wednesdays throughout the year.

Overlooking this huge square is the King's Head Inn, over the door of which, in faded lettering, are the words:

EXCISE OFFICE
.LICENSED TO LET POST HORSES

—

POST HORSES

It conjures up the animated scene prior to 1850 when the Inn was a posting house – horses hired and changed on one's journey, and post chaises being hired and making their way to Ripon and Knaresborough across the bridge. To reach the latter, we go along Silver Street to join the main road between Ripon and Leyburn, then down to the crossing of the Ure, a sizeable river here, leaving the town high and dry above the water even in times of extreme flood.

Here is a really well-built, beautifully-cut mellow stone structure with neverending traffic, heavy and light. There is little chance to stand and dream on this bridge even in the niches above the cutwaters, unless it be late at night in the summer or early evening in the winter. The nicer side from an elegant and artistic point of view is upstream. It consists of four almost semi-circular arches. The downstream side was widened subsequent to complete rebuilding and regrettably has lost some of its former beauty. It is massive rather than artistic, and looks as it would stand no nonsense from the river, no matter how flooded it may be. Its parapet bears the date 1754 – that is when the old wooden structure was dismantled following many years of constant repairs, something like two centuries after Leland visited it. Subsequent widening added about one-third of the present width.

Our old friend, Leland, visited Masham, and some 28 years after his death the sum of £15 was spent on repairs. In 1614 and 1647 the sum of £40 was spent on repairs on each occasion, but in 1665 a major repair cost £400, and following further repairs over a period of 70 years, the bridge was taken down and completely rebuilt in stone. Pending completion, it is said that a footbridge and a ferry boat were used for crossing.

Care must be taken after crossing the bridge from the town as there is an immediate T junction – left for Thornton Stewart and right for Aldburgh Hall, West Tanfield and Ripon. At this point it is interesting to note what Leland said:

> 'Masseham has a praty quik market town and a fair
> Chirch, an a bridge of tymbre, a little beynethe
> Masseham on the other side of Yore ryver lye the Aldbury
> village. At the end of Masseham townlet, I passed
> over a fair ryver called Bourne, it goeth into the Ure
> thereby a little byneth the bridge'.

Note the different ways of spelling the main river. The Bourne, incidentally, is now spelled Burn.

Let us now retrace our steps into the market place and take the Swinton Road, crossing the river Burn by a stone bridge which divides the golf course into two parts, and make our way to two unique bridges. Passing the castle's main entrance, we turn right until we meet with an extraordinary scene, Quarry Gill on the Swinton Estate.

The Danby family became Lords of the Manor through the marriage of Geoffrey Scrope's daughter to Sir Christopher Danby. This was early in the 16th century when there was no male heir of the Scrope family. Many generations later the man of business, a good benefactor and responsible for many innovations, was William Danby. One particular innovation was the

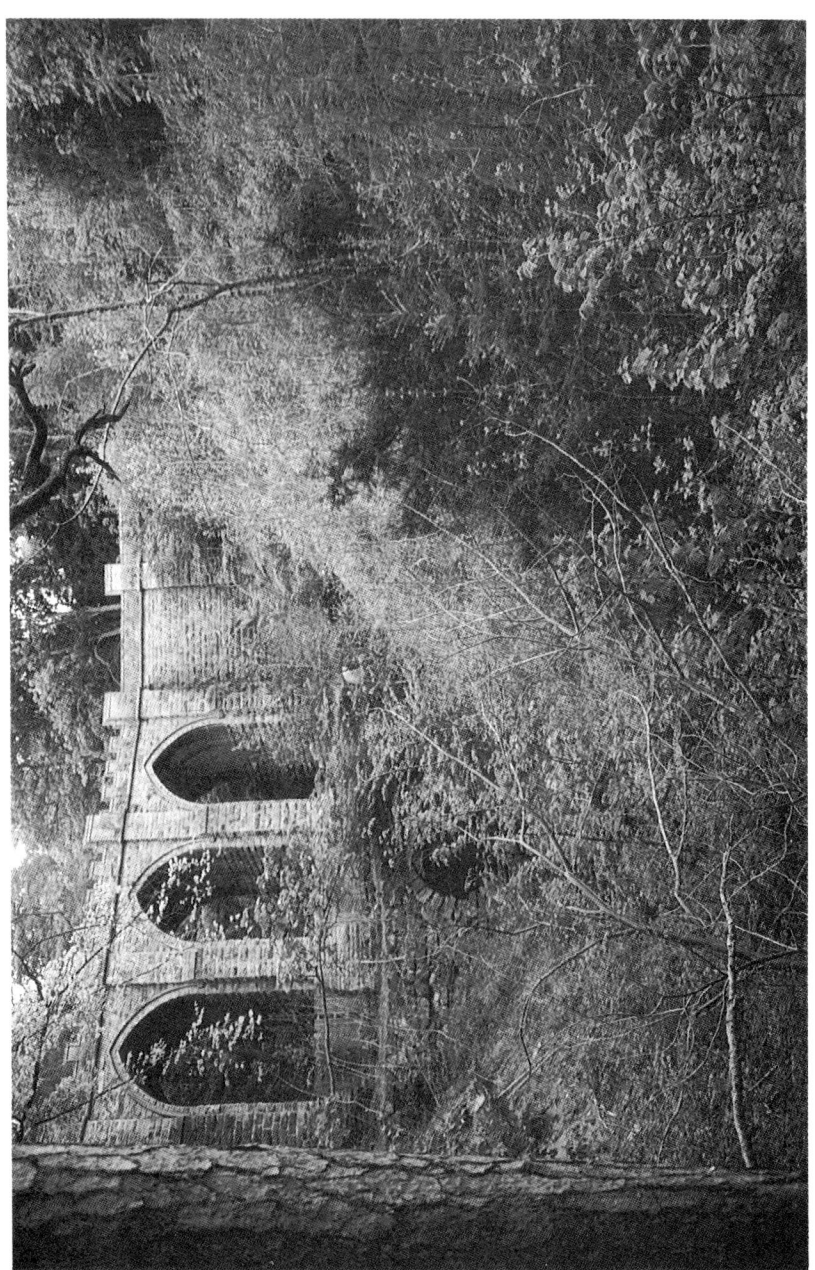

The bridge at Swinton

avoidance of a very steep and difficult crossing of Quarry Gill. This hazard he overcame by building a new bridge over the Gill. It consists of three very high pointed arches with battlemented parapets. The view downstream is of the well-wooded, almost breathtaking ravine leading to the Burn valley with the villages of Healey and Fearby on the far side. Upstream, the scene is quite different – rhododendrons and huge shrubs as well as stately trees fill the steep sides of the gill at the bottom of which gurgles the beck. At the north end of the bridge is a stone gazebo with an inscription which reads:

THIS SEAT OVERLOOKING SOME OF THE BEAUTIFUL WORKS
OF THE CREATOR WAS BUILT WITH GRATEFUL MIND BY
WILLIAM DANBY ESQ AD 1832

The bridge's special interest lies in the fact that its piers stand on top of the old packhorse bridge far down below. The latter consists of a single stone arch and at present has no parapets. Both ends curve round to the north and the tracks leading from them disappear into the steep sides of the V-shaped valley. The soil of the latter must have washed down over the years and covered the approach tracks which wound their way round the hillsides. The battlemented bridge was built in 1832, and descending to have a close look at the packhorse bridge needs great care. One side of the gill is quite a jungle, but the other side is quite clear of growth except for the boles of mature beech trees.

One wonders how the little packhorse bridge, which is quite wide, supports the great weight of those tall piers of the 'modern' bridge. A view of the former, before 1832, inspired the late George Cuitt, an artist, who found Masham to his liking and made it his home. The little bridge itself makes one realize the great skill of its builders.

We cannot leave this attractive area without having a look at another creation of William Danby – the Druid's Temple at Ilton, only a mile or so from Quarry Gill. Near the water splash on the road from Healey, one turns left up the hill. A large plantation on the right-hand side is followed, and soon an entrance with rustic tables and seats is reached. A good track through the trees leads to a surprising sight. Mr Danby's staff were apparently short of work due to crop failure, and to keep them employed he gave them the job of quarrying large quantities of stone to build the temple, which is reminiscent of Stonehenge. This was in about 1800.

RIPON

On our way downstream, we pass over West Tanfield Bridge, with the famous view from the west parapet of the Marmion Tower and Church. The bridge is massive if not artistic, but for one which is said to have had no less than 17 arches, we must visit the North Bridge at Ripon. It is a very long and level one, so much so that many motorists hardly notice that they are going along a bridge at all.

Although we are encouraged to 'stay awhile' in Ripon and rightly so, we must press on to the bridge. Among the very many and varied attractions of Ripon, there is one which cannot fail to intrigue the visitor. The blowing of the horn by the Wakeman at 9 o'clock every evening throughout the year has been a tradition for over a thousand years. Householders and tradesmen paid 2d per annum, in respect of each door of the property they occupied, and in return, after 9 o'clock, the Wakeman and the Mayor were responsible for goods stolen from the property. Surely one of the first forms of insurance?

The little river Laver is crossed when entering the city from the south, and the Market Place is reached by means of two very narrow streets, but the bridge which takes us out of Ripon to the Great North Road and the plain of York lies immediately to the east of the city.

Today, it is difficult to see all 17 arches at the North Bridge but the river Ure flows through six of them at a little more than average level. On the south end there are three more visible. At the north end more arches are in evidence and steel supports under the approach roads can be seen. The ancient part is largely at the north end, and on the downstream side most of the arches are slightly pointed, but the arch at midstream is the most attractive of them all. It has a very decided point, and a set of 10 stone corbels appear to help to support the parapet; this feature is absent from the rest. Looking under these arches, it is quite apparent that widening has taken place over the years on two separate occasions. On the upstream side all the arches, which are segmental, are rounded. The cutwaters both upstream and down are pointed and slope down from well below the parapets, so there are no niches from which to view the water, but there is, of course, a sidewalk on both sides of the carriageway.

At the south end there is an historic line carved in the stonework showing the extraordinarily high watermark on the occasion of a flood on 29th January 1883, when the low-lying ground, particularly at that end, would have been several feet under water. All the arches would then be coping, but only just, with the abnormal conditions.

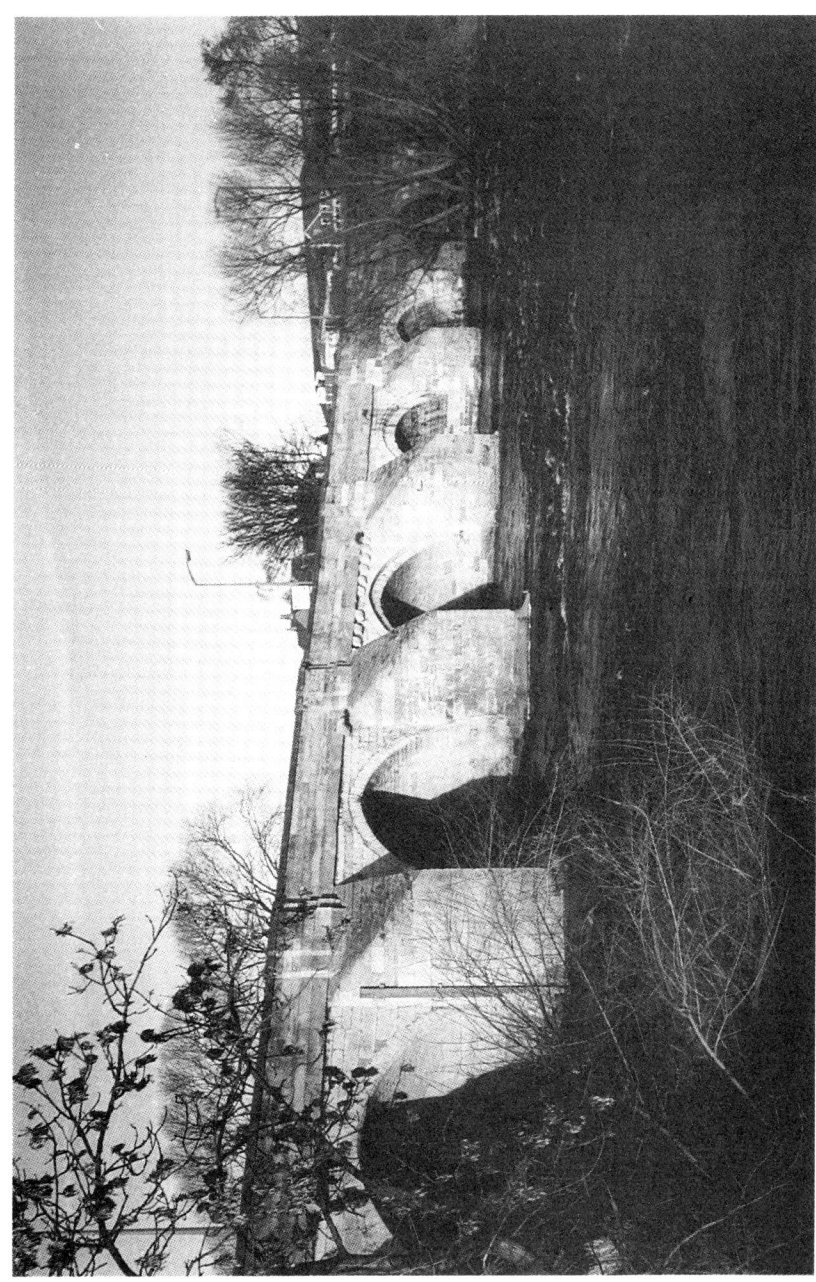

The North Bridge at Ripon

A bridge was in evidence here in the late 13th century, and early in the 14th century tolls were exacted to pay for upkeep, but in 1365 it was alleged that some of the toll money was being used for other purposes. Appropriate action was taken, an auditor being appointed to examine the records.

By 1608, like so many other bridges, Ripon's North Bridge was in a parlous state, and both the North and West Ridings contributed to the cost of repairs over a period of about 100 years.

Before that time, the indefatigable Leland had a look and said it had seven arches, so little change has taken place since the 16th century. He referred, of course, to the number of arches under which the Ure would flow at that time. It is easy to visualize the build-up of sand and silt over the years on the south bank upstream, where the arches are now normally free of flowing water. At the north end of the bridge, the river has eaten its way into the bank and water trickles through the arch which would formerly be on dry land.

A remarkable bridge, and in some ways comparable with Wakefield. Oh, that it had a chantry chapel, like the latter. Even with today's heavy traffic, it copes admirably, and so one cannot visualize a concrete or steel structure as a bypass. In fact, the days of steel have long since gone with the passing of the once-nearby railway bridge.

BOROUGHBRIDGE

If we approach Boroughbridge from the south, we see the Great North Road cross the Aire at Ferrybridge, and the old Roman road to the north cross the same river at Castleford. Having crossed the Wharfe at Tadcaster, and the Nidd at Cattal, by the Roman road (as far as possible) we arrive at Boroughbridge, or rather a little south of it, because we cannot fail to stop at Aldburgh, and its adjacent Roman town Isurium. Aldburgh has a lovely village green, at the top of which you enter the site, which is full of Roman remains. First is the small but fascinating museum where you pay your dues. Then the remains of the town walls come into view, and the forum and temple stones, all in red sandstone. The musts for all visitors are the two mosaic floors, well-protected by brick and stone walls and roof. They are viewed through windows, or through a wide-meshed grilled door. They are perfect, except for one, which has a concrete repair job which only slightly detracts from the handiwork. The whole area is under the care of English Heritage. Turning left at the foot of the green to reach Boroughbridge itself, a tall cross about 18 feet high can be seen on a triangle of green. Hard by is the restored Old Manor House, half-timbered. The cross was originally erected in the Market Place at Boroughbridge to commemorate the Battle of that town, but has stood in Aldburgh for some 140 years.

Although Aldburgh was occupied by the Romans, it continued as a civil settlement under them as it did when established originally by the Brigantes.

The river Ure, some 1200 yards away, needed to be crossed and so Boroughbridge came about with its Pons Burgi. On our way to it we cannot fail to note St James' Square, the quaint side streets, antique shops, hotels and, in particular, The Crown. The church is modern, but contains many relics of the former building.

The importance of Boroughbridge grew with the passing of the centuries. The Great North Road was its main thoroughfare and made its way over the river. The road from Ripon to York came this way; river traffic found the town a convenient stopping-place, or even a terminus for large ships. Turning the corner at the Crown Hotel, the way down to the river lies ahead with the bridge of bridges. A crossing of some sort has existed for something like 2000 years, but records show that the Normans built a wooden bridge – it was certainly made of timber when, during the Battle of Boroughbridge, a Welshman hid himself under the bridge. When the Earl of Hereford, a supporter of Lancaster, was attempting to storm it with his men, the Welshman thrust his spear through a gap and badly wounded the Earl, who fell forward. Lancaster, in spite of a final effort to ford the river, failed to do so and was eventually led to the block at Pontefract, of all places, because the castle there was his own. He was summarily condemned to death as a traitor in June 1322, led out of town on an old horse without a bridle, and duly executed.

After crossing the bridge from the south to Kirby Hill, one comes almost immediately upon the bloodstained battleground, where, some 500 years later, many relics were unearthed, such as pieces of armour, swords and bones.

Boroughbridge received its Charter as a borough in 1557. Hostelries and stabling had become part of Boroughbridge which had become an important coaching centre. Farriers and wheelwrights came and set up their stalls, and, with the coming of the canal in 1770, the town's activity knew no bounds. One can easily imagine the loading and unloading of all manner of goods near that old bridge. Then came the railway, and the old character of the town largely disappeared, but eventually, with the coming of the internal combustion engine, the character changed again and Boroughbridge once more became a stopping place for travellers, both for tourists and business people. By 1965 the motor traffic became a great problem, and the Great North Road bypassed the town. Fears that the place would become a ghost town were soon dispelled as travellers actually left the bypass to visit the town's many attractions.

The bridge is best seen in the morning sunshine from downstream, but even so the massive widening has spoiled the picture, and on the upstream side the ancient aspect of the bridge is completely lost. The ancient pointed arches have long since disappeared from view. Pons Burgi, as it was originally known, was made of stone some years before John Leland visited it in the 16th century. No doubt he felt that it was in a ruinous state, because in 1632, and during the next 100 years, there was a constant repair bill. Before the original widening took place in the 18th century, the story goes that two wagons met and, in the course of endeavouring to pass each other, one of them caused the parapet to give way, and one wagon fell, in the most undignified way, into the river.

To settle the state of affairs since 1562, one has only to look at the stone plaque on the upstream parapet, which reads:

BOROUGHBRIDGE
Downstream side built 1562
Upstream side built 1784
Widened and reconstructed
1949

Who is going to dispute that?

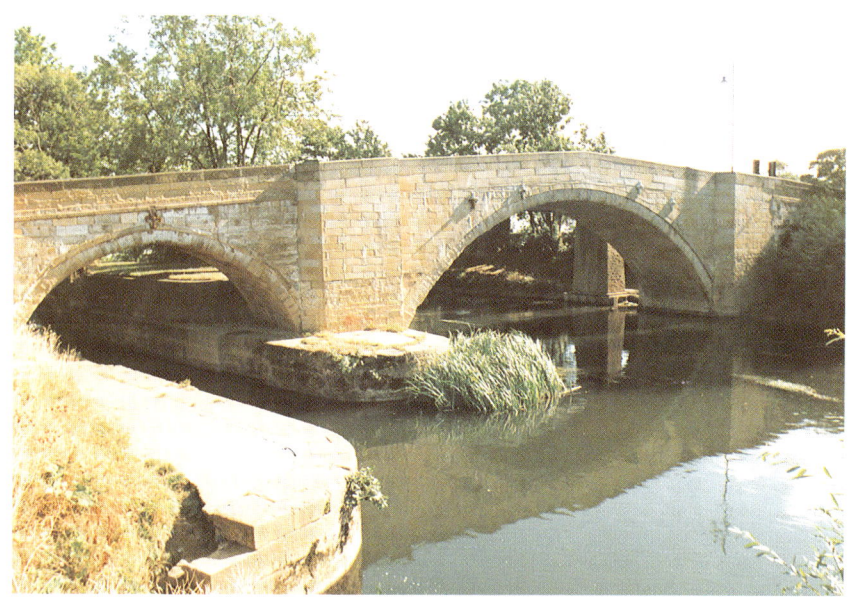

Stamford Bridge

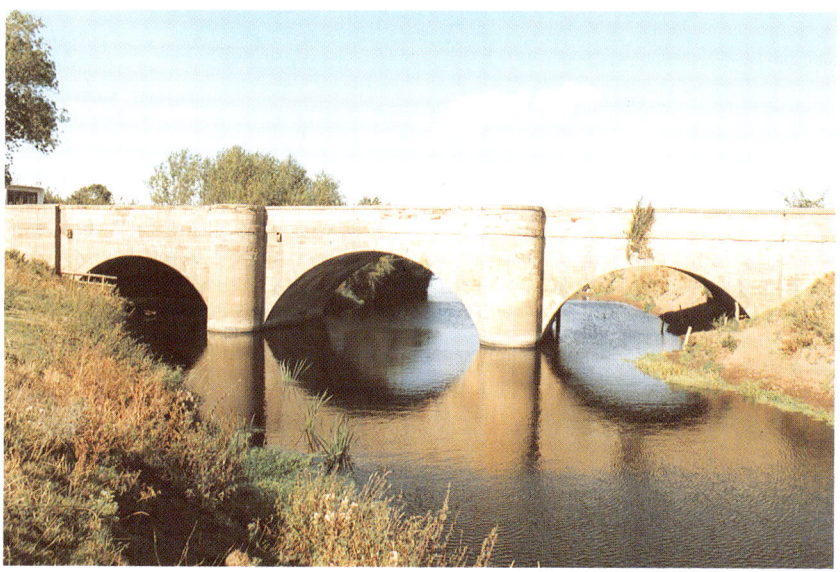

Skip Bridge

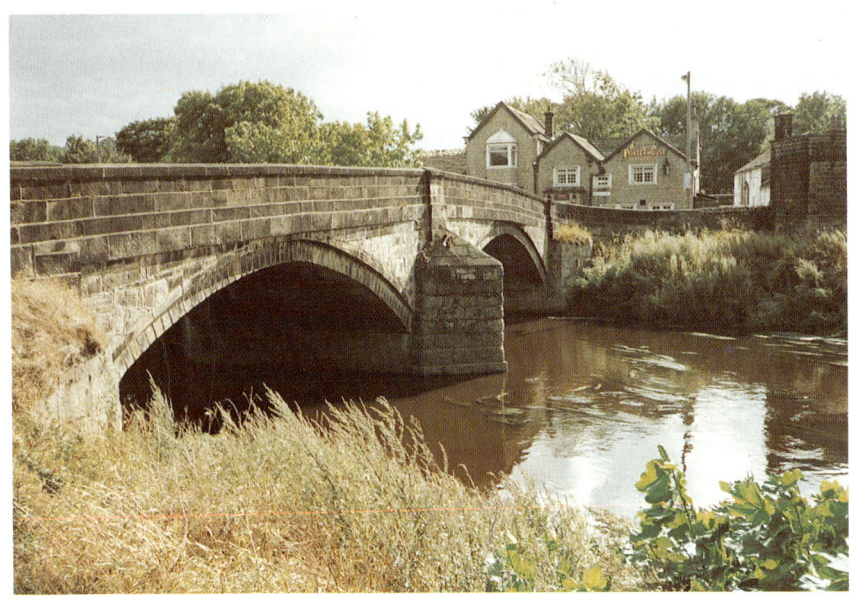

Apperley Bridge and George and Dragon

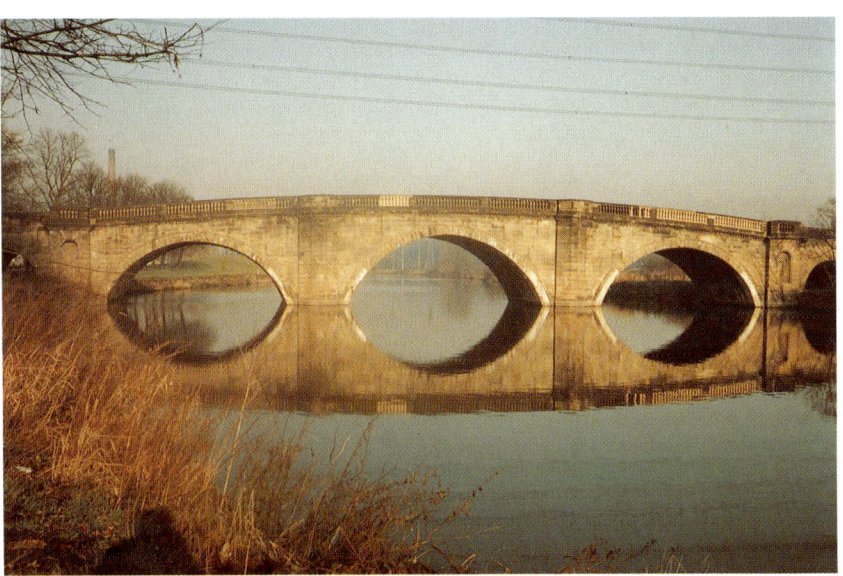

Ferrybridge

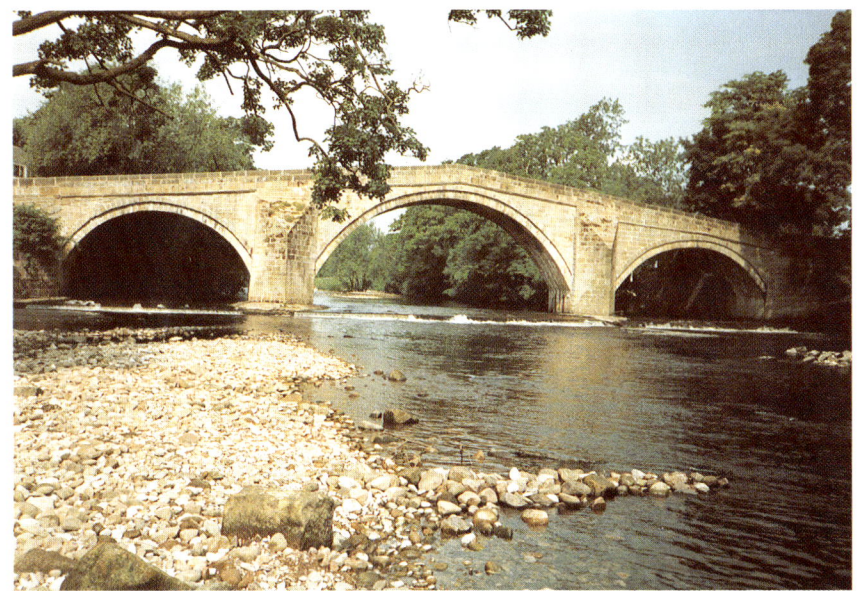

Ilkley Old Bridge

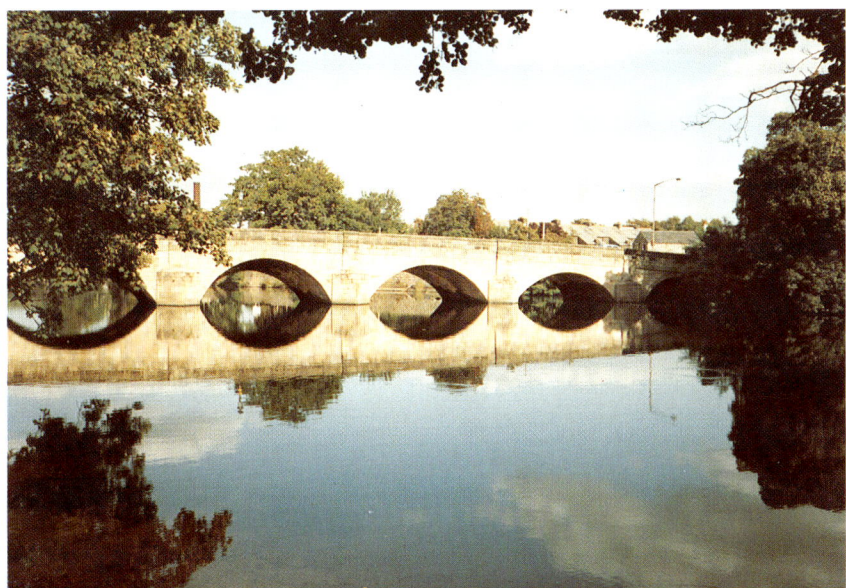

Otley Bridge

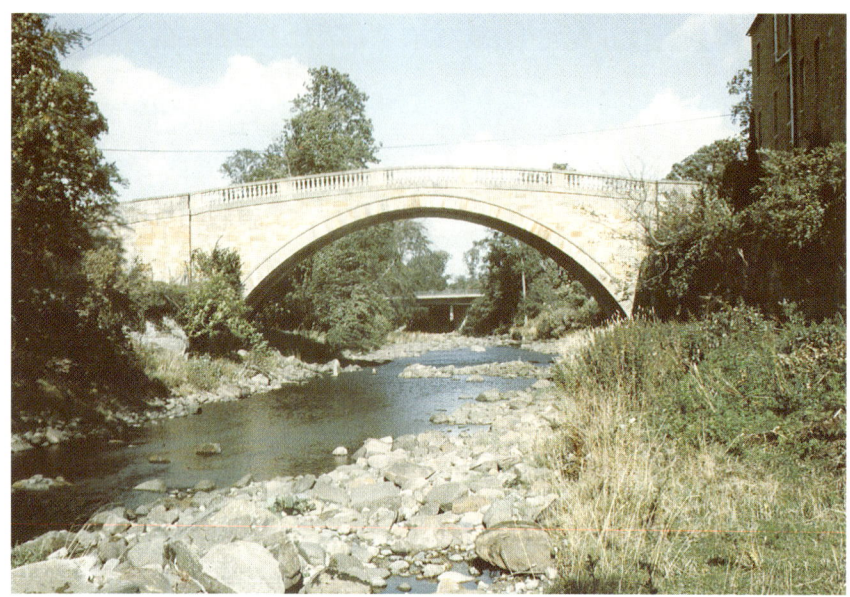

Greta Bridge

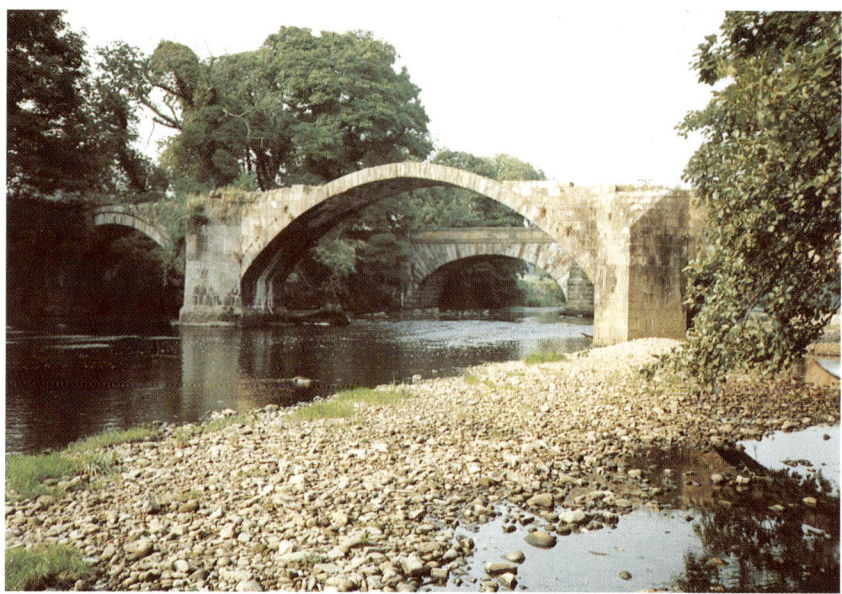

Cromwell's Bridge

THE RIVER OUSE

Of all the English rivers flowing into the North Sea, the Humber and the Thames both have broad estuaries which lead a long way inland and gave access, in the past, to a wide area by ship. In Yorkshire, we are concerned with the Ouse, which pours its waters into the Humber. As the Ouse is tidal, being awash with the incoming tide from the Humber, it is not surprising that York became a great centre, both militarily and tradewise, from at least Roman times.

As the Ure merges with the Ouse a short distance downstream from Boroughbridge, we must follow the latter river and have a peep at York. However, there is so much to see and talk about in that ancient city that we will confine our attention to some of the bridges over the Ouse and the Foss, which enters the main river near Castle Mills Bridge. Foss Bridge, whilst comparatively small, has considerable charm and reflects the classical style prevalent some 180 years ago. It has one arch with balustraded parapets, easily seen from the metal bridge at the lower end of Piccadilly, and, for a close-up view, from the garden of the Merchant Adventurers' Hall. To stand and lean over the parapets, one must turn left after crossing the metal bridge; an ancient street – Fossgate – leads us from the bridge back to the city centre.

The bridge of bridges in York must surely be Ouse Bridge, the only crossing of the river at one time. From the city centre it is approached by means of Low Ousegate and, to obtain a good view of it, we descend the stone steps on the downstream side to King's Staith. It has three huge segmental arches with very low cutwaters which are blunt-ended; an elegant structure but with a slight hump in the middle. Turn about and look downstream and Skeldergate Bridge comes into view. This marks the end of the extant city wall, which does not reappear until Fishergate Postern Tower is reached, a little distance away. From the north parapet of Ouse Bridge looking upstream, one has a splendid view of Lendal Bridge, its steel spanning the river with some majesty. The latter gives easy access to the Minster from the huge railway station, the road passing under an arch in the city wall en route. Prior to the erection of the bridge in 1863, a ferry was the means of crossing at this point.

Ouse Bridge replaced, in 1810, an ancient crossing, or rather several crossings, the first of which existed in the 12th century. This was probably a wooden one, but it collapsed in 1154, in which catastrophe Archbishop William of York just escaped death. He died some little time after, however, and was canonized. His memory is perpetuated in a great window in the

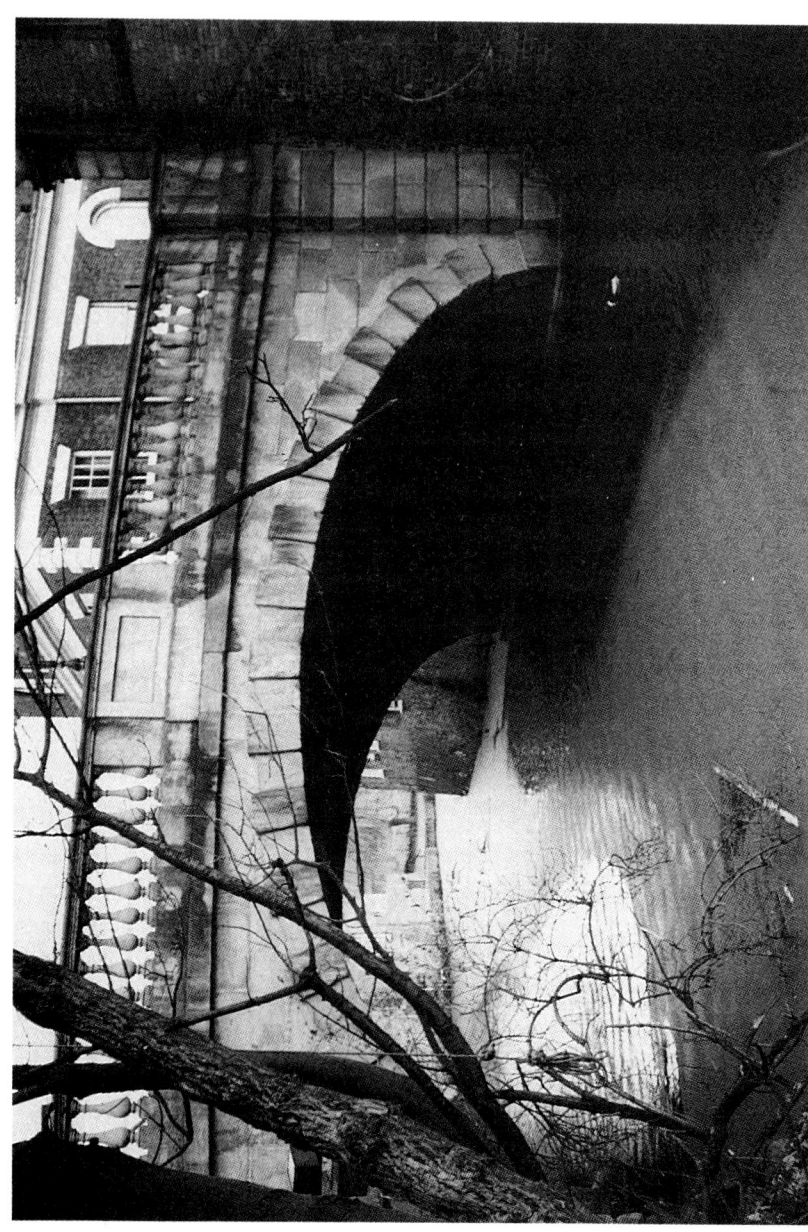

Foss Bridge in York

north choir transept of the Minster. He is shown, among very many incidents in his life, riding a white horse over Ouse Bridge. In fact, the window is known as the St William Window and rises to a great height. St William is also remembered through the lovely building known as St William's College, erected in 1460 near the Minister.

The bridge was, of course, rebuilt following the disaster, and boasted many buildings both public and private: houses, shops, a toll booth and a chapel dedicated to St William. In 1565, this bridge collapsed. It seems that the great weight of buildings, combined with flood waters containing huge blocks of ice, proved too much. As a result, a major repair job was necessary, the number of arches being reduced to five in the process. Our old friend, Leland, does not appear to record that the bridge was in a ruinous state; he did, however, go as far as to say that it has six arches, but that was before his death in 1552 and before the second disaster.

It is interesting to note that King Henry VII paid a visit to York in 1486 and was received with due pomp and ceremony on the bridge itself.

NIDDERDALE

The Nidd, for the most part, is a shy river. In its infancy, it allows itself to be swallowed by two large reservoirs, Angram and Scar House. When the dam for the latter was built, soon after World War I, for the Bradford Corporation, it was the largest in Europe. Having been released from that, the Nidd soon allows itself to be swallowed up by a limestone pothole which takes it underground for a mile or so. Even when it emerges from a cave under the road from Lofthouse to Ramsgill, it does so quietly and runs down the valley, only to be seen for a short distance before it reaches Ramsgill via a delightful little bridge. Thereafter, it is quickly swallowed up by Gowththwaite reservoir. Even after flowing over the Gowthwaite dam it hides itself at the bottom of a partially-wooded valley until it shows itself at Wath Bridge. After that it is only seen again just before it reaches Pateley Bridge. After that, only rare glimpses are seen by the motorist at Summerbridge and Warsill, until Birstwith is reached. However, between Pateley and Birstwith the river was put to much use, years ago, because it was the scene of industry in a quiet but prosperous way. Nidd water provided water power and steam power.

Just before reaching Birstwith from Darley, a tiny lane leads one down to a gem of a bridge. It is called New Bridge, and, although being comparatively unknown to the average traveller, it is on the Nidderdale Way. Even the latter leaves the river at this point and wanders off 'over the hills and far away.' It is called New Bridge, as it was almost completely rebuilt in 1822. It was a packhorse affair and packhorses on their way from Swarcliffe to Hartwith heralded their approach with little bells on their harness. The Nidd is of no mean width here and the single-span segmental arch spells much skill combined with beauty. On the north side, the packhorse track crosses the dismantled railway, now grass-grown, and takes one up the hill, crossing the Pateley Bridge–Ripley road on its way to the north-east towards Fountains Abbey and Ripon.

The bridge is one which few photographers can pass without bringing out their cameras. The immediate environment fits in beautifully. The original bridge was certainly in use as far back as 1594, and it is thought that, in the early monastic days, a bridge existed a little downstream possibly coinciding with the Monks Wall, which stretched from the river to Fountains Abbey, and marked the boundary of the abbey lands. The footpath which starts just west of Burnt Yates village follows the site of the Monks Wall for part of the way to the river, but leaves it about halfway, turning right and past Dunmore House to join the packhorse lane to the present bridge.

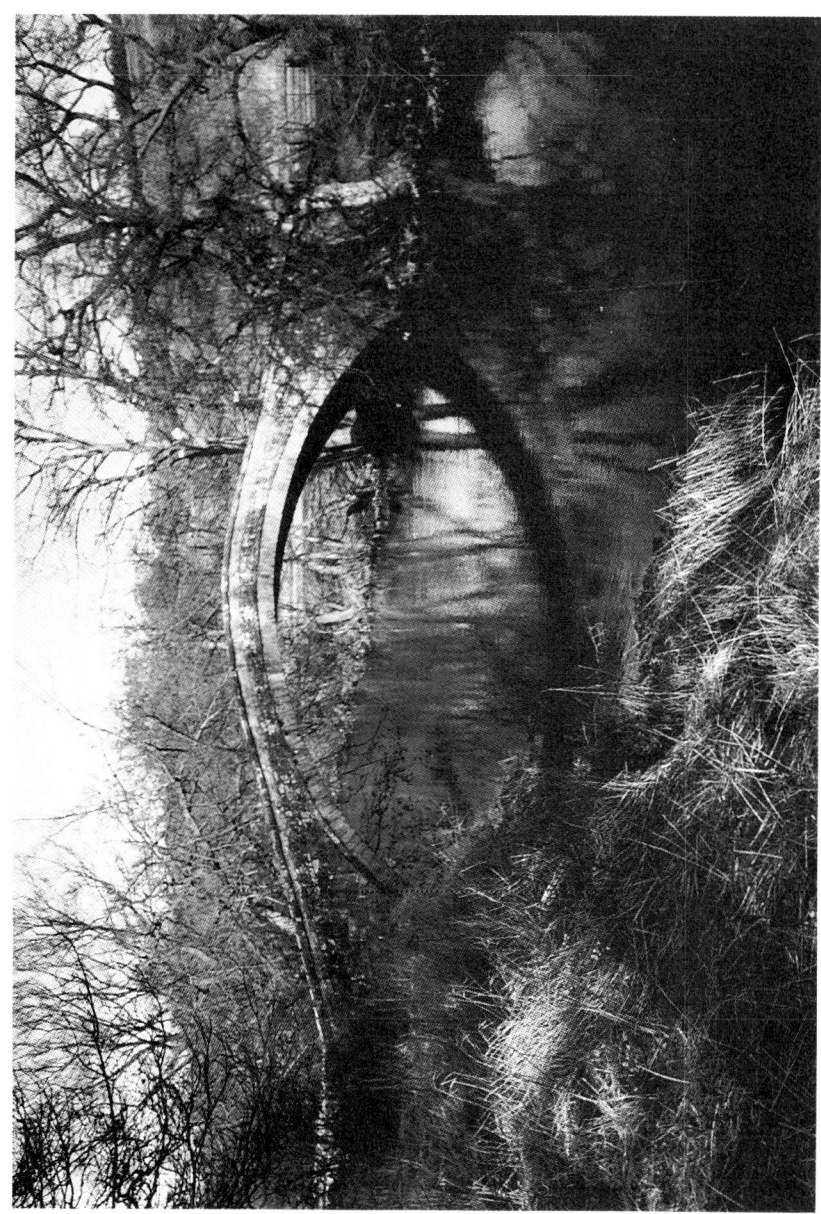

The New Bridge at Birstwith

THORNTHWAITE

Of all the little bridges, especially those which carried packhorses, Thornthwaite must surely be one of the most charming. Unfortunately, it keeps secret a great deal of its romantic history. It is situated at the foot of a narrow lane, and crosses Red Beck, a feeder of the Nidd. From whatever angle one views it, the picture is a delight. No roadway goes over it now, as it stands serene away from the present lane which bypasses it.

The ancient Forest of Knaresborough extends up this valley, and includes the bridge as well as the little church a hundred yards up the lane. The church was erected in AD 1810, dedicated to St Saviour, and is on the site of an ancient chapel. The monks passed this way when travelling from Fountains Abbey to Bolton, on an old route from Ilkley to Ripon, using the little bridge en route. Packhorses used it, too, of course.

It is interesting to note a reference to the chapel of old in the Honour of Knaresborough Court Rolls:

"(AD) 1409, Thornthwaite, ld, new rent of John Pulayn for one dariate of land of new assart (clearing) for the Chapel to be built, to hold him".

One penny, indeed!

Just downstream from the bridge, on the north-east side of the beck, is a series of numbered boundary stones. It is quite unusual to see so many still standing over such a comparatively short distance.

Nowadays, one crosses the beck, alas, by means of a flat concrete affair which will serve as a ford in the event of a serious flood. Once over the hill one reaches Dacre and the Darley en route to Birstwith.

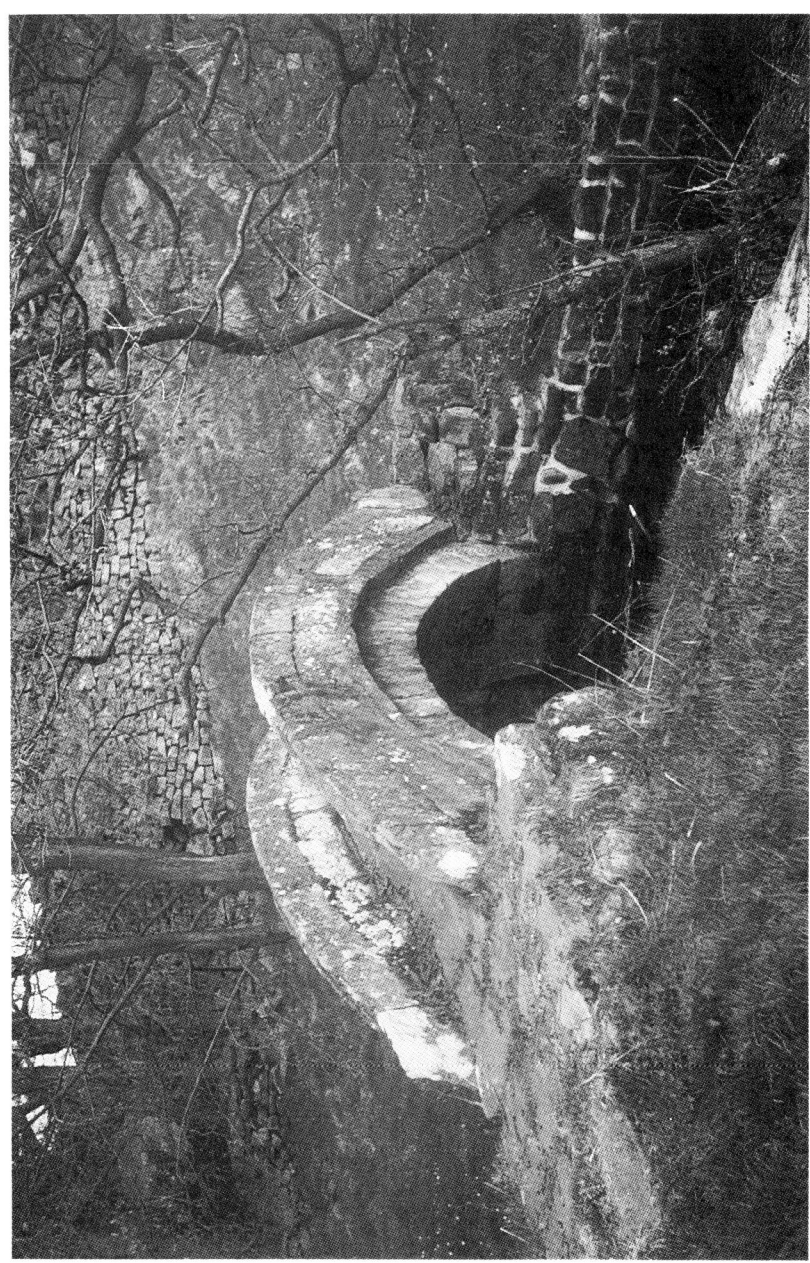

Thornthwaite Bridge

HAMPSTHWAITE

Only a few miles downstream from Birstwith is Hampsthwaite and its unique bridge.

The village dates back to Brigantian times, when it was under the jurisdiction of Aldborough (Isurium) near Boroughbridge. The Romans knew Hampsthwaite and so did the Normans, but it did not appear in the Domesday Book, probably because it came under Aldborough.

The church of St Thomas à Becket was built in 1175 and founded by one William de Stuteville. His brother-in-law, Hugh de Morecille, was associated with the murder of Thomas à Becket in 1170, and it seems likely that de Stuteville, in an endeavour to clear himself from this unfortunate episode, dedicated his church to St Thomas who was canonised in 1173. Most of the church, as it stands today, was rebuilt in 1820 and restored as recently as 1921. Among the many memorials inside is a large marble one near the font, which commemorates Amy Woodforde-Finden who is buried in the churchyard. She will be well remembered for her musical compositions, notably the Indian Love Lyrics.

Nearby is the ancient and charming bridge, which was widened in 1640 by about two feet and not widened since. There must be few bridges of such great span which remain so narrow today. It carries one-way traffic. The corbels on both the upstream and downstream side hold up the parapets which, when they were replaced, gave the bridge the extra width. The niches immediately above the cutwaters give refuge from vehicles for foot travellers. The three segmental arches of great span, and the narrowness of the carriageway, go a long way to making the bridge unique. The method of widening so many years ago by means of corbels adds to its attractive features in no small measure.

The Roman road from Ilkley to Aldborough is said to have crossed the Nidd at Hampsthwaite by means of a ford. Traces of Roman work upstream would appear to confirm this.

On leaving the north end of the bridge, it is worthwhile noting the inscribed stone in the wall, and the seat on the right-hand side. On proceeding up the hill a mile or so, we find Clint with its remains of the village stocks, mounting steps and stone pyramid on the right.

A few miles downstream is Nidd Bridge, near Ripley, after which the river enters a deep and narrow defile in the magnesian limestone belt. At Knaresborough, the defile results in the spectacular position of the town. There are three bridges here, two road bridges, and the imposing railway viaduct which figures in so many general views of Knaresborough. There is

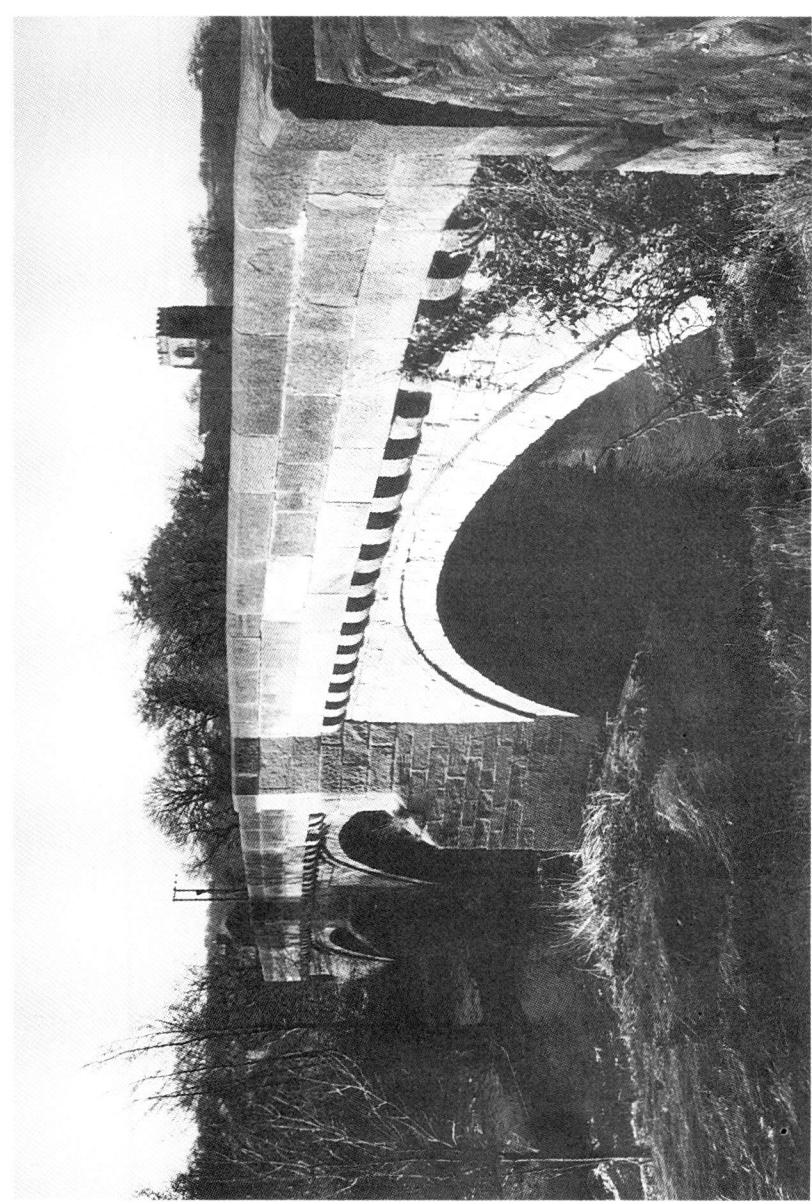

Hampsthwaite Bridge

so much to write, and indeed so much has already been written, about its many and varied attractions that we must very reluctantly press on to Walshford, Cattal and Skip Bridges where the Nidd resumes its quiet way through the meadows to join the Ouse.

Walshford is an ancient crossing of the Great North Road over the river. Nearby is the Bridge Inn. Greatly enlarged, the Inn now seems to face the other way, whilst the old road peters out just past the lodge gates.

There was a bridge at Walshford early in the 13th century, and in Henry III's time there was a corn mill here, as well as at Hunsingore just east of the North Road. It seems likely that the Knights Templar erected the bridge and kept it in repair. Before 1240, weekly markets were held at Walshford every Tuesday as well as a four-day fair held at Midsummer. The Templars were established a little upstream from Walshford at Ribston; the order of these military friars was established in England in the 12th century and came to Ribston a few years later, and thence to Hunsingore.

There was a chapel on or very near the bridge at Walshford, but it is thought that it did not survive the Dissolution, when the bridge was rebuilt.

Walshford, being on the Great North Road, would, like Ferrybridge, Wetherby and Boroughbridge, be a favourite stopping place in the coaching days. Scotch cattle would come lumbering along, footsore and weary, and there would be hold-ups of impatient coach drivers. The sound of champing of bits and the clatter of hooves would fill the air with somewhat profane shouts to add to the confusion.

To have a look at the bridge, one must go down the old north road at the side of the Inn and, after passing the lodge gates, push one's way through nettles and bushes. Down below is the Nidd, quietly pursuing its course, and the modern section of the A1 crossing it in one fell swoop. Huge concreted square pillars support the carriageway, but there is one redeeming feature – large segmental arches span the river as part of the whole structure. Alas, they are made of concrete, and replace an ancient bridge of four arches.

So now we take the flyover from Walshford and very shortly reach the timberyard, just before the road rises up to the church of St John the Baptist at Hunsingore. Here the key to the church can be obtained. Built in 1868, the church replaced an ancient one nearby which was pulled down. The large yard, which is entered through a curious four-arched stone erection, contains the tombstone of John Goodricke, the well-known astronomer who died in 1786, a member of the famous family of that name.

At Hunsingore, where a crossing of the Nidd once existed, is a mound near the river associated with the establishment of the Knights Templars. The bridge was never rebuilt, but a footbridge, which can be seen from the mound, spans the water, and is used by anglers from Harrogate and Bradford.

Leaving this quiet village, the road leads to the east and in a short while we reach Cattal and its bridge.

CATTAL BRIDGE

One's first impression of the bridge, and indeed the river Nidd which flows beneath, is its comparative smallness. It is hard to believe that this is the Nidd, after its many wanderings so near to its unobtrusive end at Nun Monkton, where it joins the Ouse. The water is quite deep, however, and quite still.

If one had followed the Roman crossing some 1900 years ago, the bridge would have been a little lower downstream at perhaps a shallower and wider part. This would have led to one straight up the little main street of Cattal, instead of making a detour as at present. It is said that a ford was in existence at the time of Henry III (1216–1272). The river is banked to prevent flooding. About 100 years ago, blocks of ice about a ton in weight were brought down with the flood waters, but our little bridge apparently survived the onslaught, and the village blacksmith's hammers were used to break up the blocks. Some 150 years ago, a similar flood brought down huge blocks of ice which broke down the bridge at Hunsingore, one mile upstream. The present bridge at Cattal consists of three segmental arches of stone, with pointed cutwaters which rise, to the top of the parapets, and presents an attractive picture. It is about 200 years old – a surprising little structure.

The village has no church, but if, after coming down the main street of the village, one avoids crossing the bridge, Hunsingore with its ancient church comes into view. Here lived Colonel Thornton, who raised the Yorkshire Blues against the Young Pretender in the 18th century. He later bought Allerton Mauleverer mansion, and the famous Blind Jack of Knaresborough himself, dressed in blue and buff, acted as a recruiting sergeant. He raised no less than 150 men and joined the Colonel on his march to Scotland.

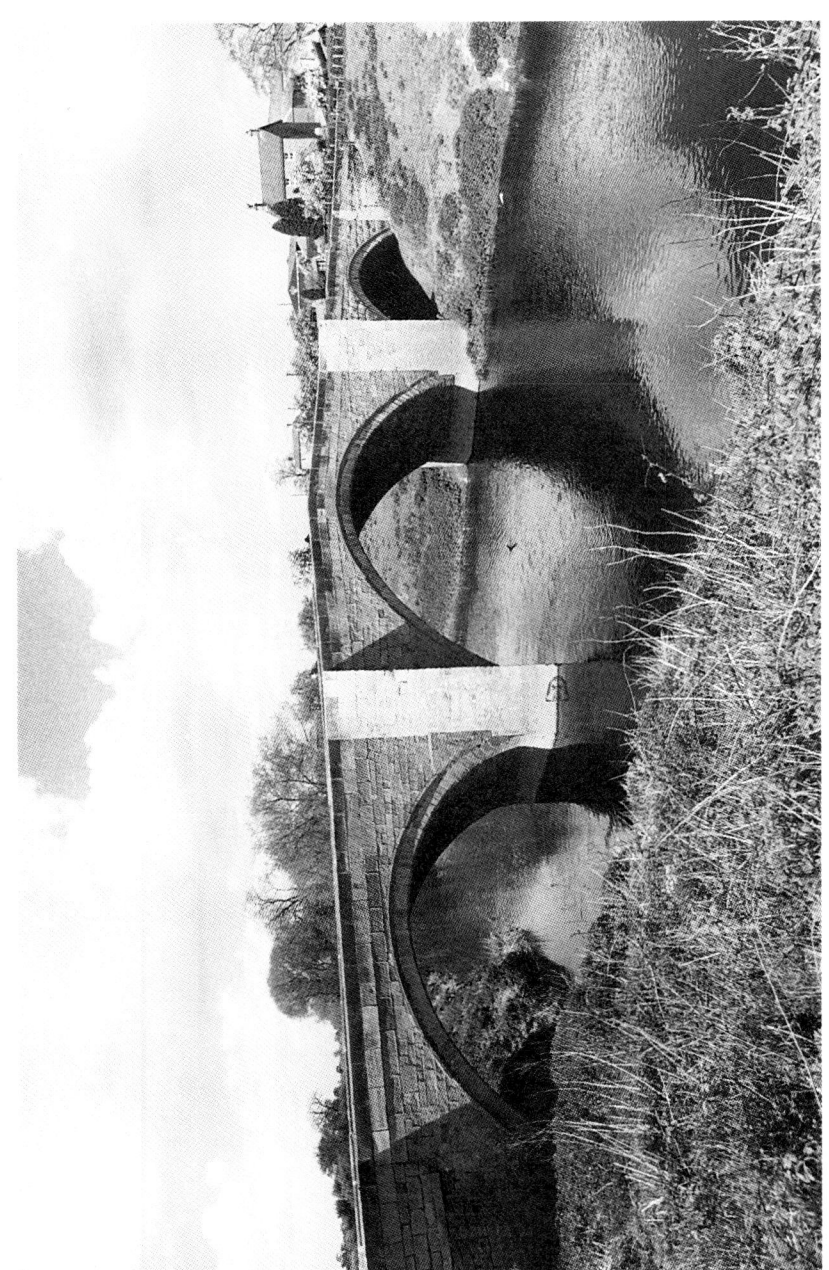

The bridge at Cattal

SKIP BRIDGE

This stands on the old road from Knaresborough to York. One cannot fail to associate this three-arched bridge of mellow stone with the nearby site of the Battle of Marston Moor, 1644, when over 4,000 Englishmen died. The three lovely arches are separated by rounded cutwaters, and looking over the fields from the niches in the south parapet, the vast area known still as Marston Moor spreads itself into the distance. It is now, of course, a well-cultivated area and could hardly be described as a moor as it was in Leland's time, when it was wild with thistles and furze. It is said that a party of Dutchmen came over to Yorkshire c 1688 to drain and dyke the moor; the result of their work is surely evident today.

Before the Reformation, Skip Bridge was a substantial structure of timber, and a long stone causeway connected it with York. Again, we quote Leland:

> "It [the causeway] hath 19 small bridges on it for avoydinge and over-passynge carres cumming out of the mores thereby. One Blake that was twys maior of Yorke, made this causey and a nother without one of the suburbs of Yorke. This Blakeman hath a solemn obiit in the Minster of Yorke and a Cantuarie at Richmond."

The Old Skip Bridge Inn? Alas, no more, but memories of this one-time hostelry linger on. During the memorable parliamentary election for the County of York in 1807, the poll went on for two weeks. Local Inns kept open house, and the contestants spent £2,306:9:2¼d on refreshments at the Skip Bridge Inn alone. Of this sum, no less than £1,700 was spent on wine, ale and liquor. Wine especially was bestowed on the electorate, which was regarded by some, even in those days, as an evil practice. It was on this occasion that the famous William Wilberforce was elected, along with Lord Milton, against the Hon H Lascelles. The building, a red brick double-fronted house, is now a farm occupied by Mr John Barnes, and faces the modern road, although it stands back a little. It was a coaching inn dating back to 1690, and inside it still retains some of the old features. Mr Barnes possesses a photograph of the building with the inn sign over the door, said to have been taken in the year 1900. Mounting steps adjacent to an outbuilding are still to be seen. Curiously enough, the former inn is something approaching half a mile east of the Bridge, on slightly higher ground, maybe to avoid being flooded. That part of the Slingsby estate (Red House) on which the building stands was sold in 1916 to a teetotaller, who sought to close the inn, and eventually in 1919 the licence lapsed.

If the sun is not shining, it is not easy to decide which is north or south of the Nidd, unless one is familiar with landmarks, because the river winds through the meadows and arable land in an astonishing way to reach, eventually, the Ouse at Nun Monkton, a very ancient village dating from Saxon times. A nunnery was established here in the 12th century, and since then the village has scarcely changed its shape; the green of 18 acres is one of the largest in England, with a huge duck pond in the middle. Near the Ouse stands the old church of St Mary at the end of a lovely treelined avenue. Even at Nun Monkton, the Nidd is still shy and needs to be sought out. It quietly glides between its high banks into the Ouse where the latter forms a surprisingly large sheet of water of several acres. To reach this, one must leave the church gates, turn to the right, and follow the Priory wall down a grassy lane.

Back on the Knaresborough road, one wonders how many times that extraordinary man, Blind Jack Metcalf of Knaresborough (1717–1818), crossed Skip Bridge and called at the inn on his many travels. He assisted the military, did horse dealing, road and bridge building, to name but some of his activities. he would surely need to use Skip Bridge to cross the Nidd, but considering his imagination and application one can picture him swimming, if not riding his horse across the water if need be. Kirk Hammerton, on the old road to Knaresborough, not far from Skip Bridge, must have also been the scene of his many travels. The church here is extraordinary, for a complete third of it is Saxon and forms a little church in itself. The remaining two-thirds is a Victorian alteration of an older structure. The Saxon part consists of a square tower, a small nave and a chancel. The whole is approached through a lychgate and up a steep path lined with yew trees. A fascinating place indeed.

Meanwhile, the approach road to Skip Bridge both from east and west seems to be a rest haven for motorists and van drivers, whilst to the north vehicles of all descriptions fly to and fro over the modern by-pass bridge, and to the south, two-coach diesel trains rattle their way along their rails between Harrogate and York.

SKIRFARE BRIDGE AND ARNCLIFFE BRIDGE

To enable one to proceed up the valley of the Wharfe from Kilnsey, a crossing of the river Skirfare is necessary, unless one travels up the minor road from Conistone. The bridge, though important, is not quite so full of charm as the name suggests. The river which we are going to follow is the Skirfare which joins the Wharfe just above Kilnsey. Its waters come down a romantic valley of Amerdale, the modern name for which is Littondale, which embraces Arncliffe, Litton, Halton Gill, Foxup and Cosh.

The poet Wordsworth referred to Amerdale in 'The White Doe of Rylstone':

> '. . . Unwooed, yet unforbidden
> The white doe followed up the vale
> Up to another cottage, hidden
> In the deep fork of Amerdale.'

A better description than 'the deep fork of Amerdale' is hard to find.

Three miles up this lovely valley is Arncliffe, the location of early scenes of the TV soap opera 'Emmerdale', and, of course, its beautiful bridge.

The beauty of Arncliffe lies in its comparatively quiet village green and the ancient houses, including the Falcon Inn, which surround it, said to be of medieval planning. In fact, the main road up the dale leaves Arncliffe just as it reaches the village, similar to East Witton where the main road leaves the village on its left. The sharp turn right leads to the church (not always as lovely as it is now) and the bridge over which the road carries on to Litton and beyond.

The bridge consists of three segmental arches, two large, and one small one on the village side. Viewed from either side it is a graceful structure and crosses a very wide stretch of river which suggests a one-time ford. It is a pity that a large tree blocks the view of the church tower which would form the background to a picture of the bridge taken from upstream. The ancient packhorse and monastic routes crossed the valley here and went over the hill to Kettlewell, and also up the valley to Litton and Halton Gill, and then over the water at Foxup.

An old story connected with Arncliffe Bridge refers to Bertha, who lived in a lowly one-roomed cottage just outside the village, and who had a reputation of foretelling future events, not always happy ones. Some 200 years ago, a young man (whom we shall call A) lived with his parents in the village, and was intrigued with Bertha, who was of uncertain age. He was

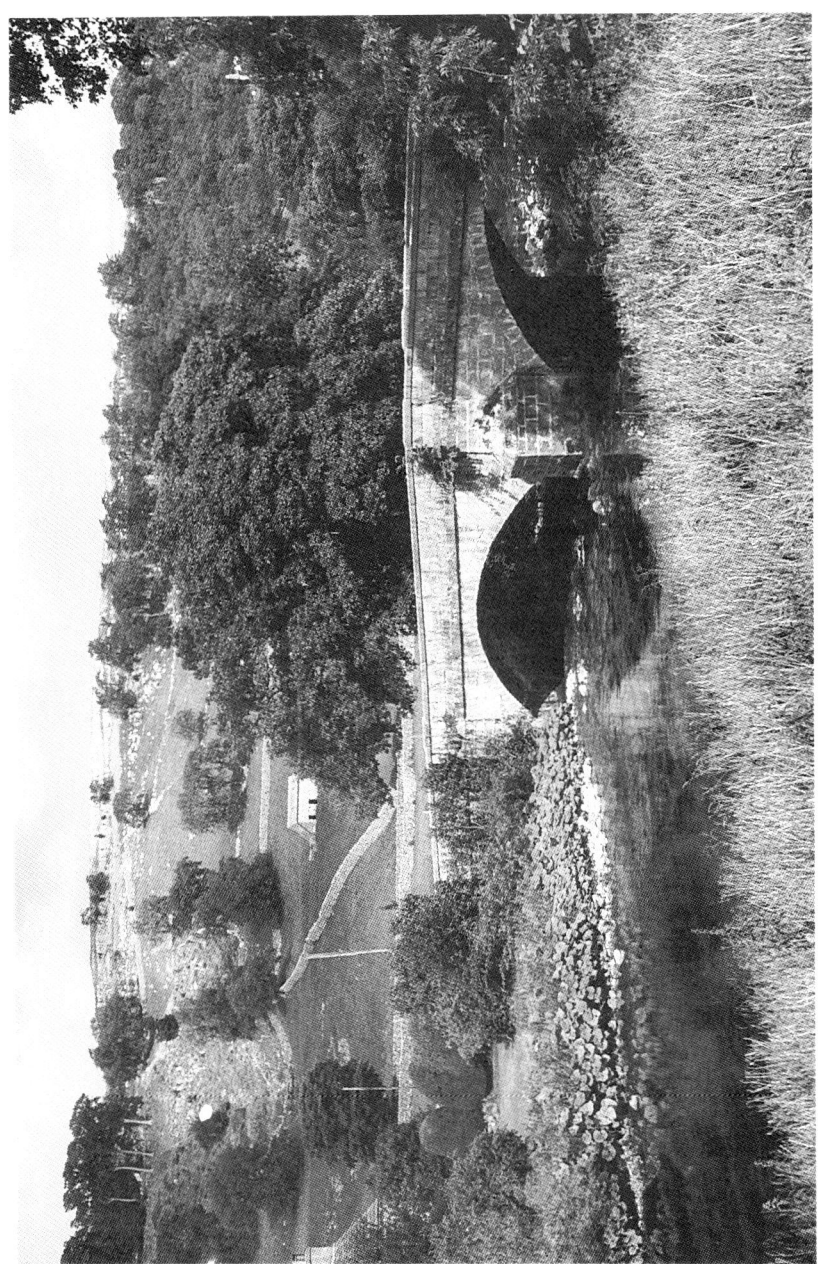

Arncliffe Bridge

led by curiosity to visit her cottage. He was welcomed, and was astonished to see Bertha seated on a three-legged stool by a turf fire, together with three black cats and a sheepdog. To her enquiry as to what she could do for him, he replied that, having seen her talking to his father about her powers, he thought he would like to see her perform some of her incantations. He said it rather naïvely, and Bertha said, "You must surely doubt my powers and consider me an impostor." He was bade to sit down and Bertha began her incantations. Into a pot of boiling water she put some odd things, bones and dried carcases of some small animals.

Looking through a glass handed to him by Bertha, he thought he saw, enveloped in the steam, the figure of a friend, who, though normally dressed, appeared pale and troubled. Bertha, having brought before him the vision of a young man known to him, bade him good night and made a request that he should go and stand on Arncliffe Bridge the following day at midnight. On questioning Bertha as to why he should do that, he was told, "Just do as I say."

After spending a restless day and evening, A repaired to Arncliffe Bridge at the appointed hour. It was a lovely night, the full moon was sailing peacefully through a cloudless sky and its beams danced on the waters of the Skirfare as it murmured under the arches of the bridge. As he stood on the parapet, soon after the church clock had struck twelve, he heard a low, moaning sound, and saw that the water was violently troubled, without any apparent cause. After a few minutes, the river became calm again, and, wondering over and over again as to what caused the disturbance, A made his way home. On his way, he came across a huge dog, apparently like a Newfoundland, which followed him, and on reaching the door, he turned round to find that the dog had disappeared. A was more intrigued than ever.

The next morning he hurried to Bertha's abode. "Well, Bertha, I obeyed you and went to the bridge at midnight."

"And to what sight were you a witness?"

"I saw nothing except a slight disturbance of the water."

"I know," Bertha said, "but did you not behold something else?"

"Nothing."

"Nothing? Your memory fails you."

"I forgot, Bertha. As I was proceeding home, I met with a Newfoundland dog, and supposed it must belong to some traveller.'

"That dog," answered Bertha, "never belonged to mortal. That dog you saw was Bargest – you may perhaps have heard of him."

"Yes, I have frequently heard tales of Bargest, but never credited them. If the legends of my native hills be true, a death may be expected to follow his appearance."

"You are right, and a death will follow last night's appearance."

"Whose death?"

"Not yours."

As Bertha refused to make any further comments, A left her, but in less than three hours he was informed that the friend, whose figure he had seen enveloped in the mist from the pot of boiling water, had that morning committed suicide by drowning himself at Arncliffe Bridge, at the very spot where a disturbance of the water had been seen.

Such is one story of the Littondale witch. Highly amusing to some, but to others a tale of dread and just one of the many legends of the past.

Before returning downstream to Skirfare Bridge, a trip up the valley from Arncliffe is worthwhile. From Halton Gill, we take a field path just across the bridge and follow the Skirfare to Foxup, where there are several little bridges, the last of which is worthy of note. It is an old packhorse affair and on a one-time route from Horton-in-Ribblesdale to the head of Littondale. It consists of a single segmental stone arch, with little more than one course of stonework immediately above it to form the roadway.

The way back to Arncliffe via Hesleden can be made on the south-west side of the valley, but in order to avoid road walking, a footbridge must be used to gain direct access to Litton. There is, however, a ford a little downstream, only to be attempted on foot after a spell of dry weather!

As a boy, having visited Arncliffe for the day, I often returned to Grassington by the mail coach – not much bigger than a trap. On the right, approaching Arncliffe Cote, the cliffs are very prominent and at the end of projecting rock makes a good profile of the Duke of Wellington.

Over Skirfare Bridge our journey takes us to Kettlewell, via its own bridge, which was extensively repaired following its partial collapse a few years ago. Five miles up the valley, passing Starbotton and Buckden, we reach our next objective, Hubberholme.

HUBBERHOLME

A feature of Hubberholme Bridge is the fact that it directly connects the Inn with the church. Not so many years ago the George Inn belonged to the church, but is still the scene of the annual letting of the 'poor pasture' upstream from the bridge. The George Inn, an ancient building in itself, was, in 1867, occupied by the parish clerk and kept as a public house, but was eventually regarded as too humble a place for the parish priest to live in, and the parsonage is now a separate building downstream.

The church is, of course, most worthy of a visit. A switch in the porch lights up the interior for ten minutes, and what an interior! There is beauty at every turn, and the rood screen, one of a few left in England, is a masterpiece of wood carving.

Ancient charm in which to say a prayer.

It seems that of all the Yorkshire Dales, Wharfedale, especially Hubberholme, whilst not as popular as Stratford-on-Avon, London or Edinburgh for example, is well and truly on the US tourist map of the British Isles. I well remember a thrilling little episode during the years just following World War II. Whilst I was in the George Inn early one Sunday afternoon with some friends, the landlord switched on the radio for all to hear the feature called 'Transatlantic Quiz'. The reader can guess our pleasure when the questioner in London asked the panel in the USA the whereabouts of Hubberholme in England. We did not have long to wait for the answer, which came loud and clear across the Atlantic:

"Would it be Wharfedale way?"

Not surprising, then, that Hubberholme 'drives Americans crazy'.

JB Priestley, the Bradford-born novelist and playwright, had similar views of Hubberholme, and chose to be remembered here. His ashes were cast here, and a plaque in the church commemorates his special love of the place. He found Hubberholme one of the smallest and most pleasant places in the world. The church of St Michael is one of the oldest buildings in Wharfedale. It existed before the abbeys of Fountains, Sawley, Kirkstall and Bolton Priory, and certainly before the Conquest.

What of the bridge? It lies on the one-time high road between Lancaster and Newcastle upon Tyne. Viewed from either side, it appears unique with its stones placed vertically, like very thin keystones, except, of course, for those in the parapets. It is a single arch affair which has stood firm for nearly 300 years. Before that, it was often in need of repair, and in 1693 it was stated to be 'in great ruin'. It was rebuilt in 1734.

YOCKENTHWAITE, CRAY AND A SERIES OF LITTLE BRIDGES

Beyond Hubberholme, the Wharfe is full of interest – one minute it is smooth and tranquil, the next it tumbles over limestone ledges and sluices itself between them. Abundant bird life adds to the charm of this portion of the modern Dales Way, which closely follows the north bank of the river. After a short two miles, we reach Yockenthwaite with its two houses standing serene and unchanging.

Just beyond is the bridge, a well-maintained, segmental, one-arched structure of wide span and substantial parapets. it is gated at the north end. As the main road up the valley – Langstrothdale – does not cross the river here, the bridge is only by local, mainly farm, traffic and walkers. Sometimes, however, motorists stop nearby and admire the bridge in its charming setting. Both the north and south ends appear to have been built up at one time to avoid a severe hump in the middle.

Yockenthwaite was on the old packhorse route from Wensleydale to Ribblesdale, on its way south via Raisgill, Horsehead Moor, Halton Gill and Foxup, and on to Horton-in-Ribblesdale and Stainforth.

Before we leave Yockenthwaite on our way to Cray, it is worth having a look at the nearby stone circle said to be of the Bronze Age.

Continuing the delightful walk from Yockenthwaite, we follow, after crossing the bridge, a well-defined path up the hill and round the back of the two houses to enjoy the views from a high level. A tiny bridge of stone with metal hand-rail is soon reached near Stans Wood, and later a footbridge over the upper reaches of Crook Gill, which cuts deeply into the limestone. The track then leads to the hamlet of Cray and the White Lion Inn, where Cray Gill, formed by a number of mountain torrents, runs at the side of the road and then under it, to present the visitor with a waterfall of admirable proportions. From the Inn we immediately follow a path down the sloping side of the valley of Cray Gill, where limestone ravines and more waterfalls follow in rapid succession, until the quaintest of quaint little stone bridges is reached just before Crook Gill joins Cray Gill. Thereafter, the path leads down to a very minor road at the west end of yet another bridge – Stubbing Bridge, a lovely old stone affair which appears to have been there from time immemorial. Turn right here for a short walk back to Hubberholme.

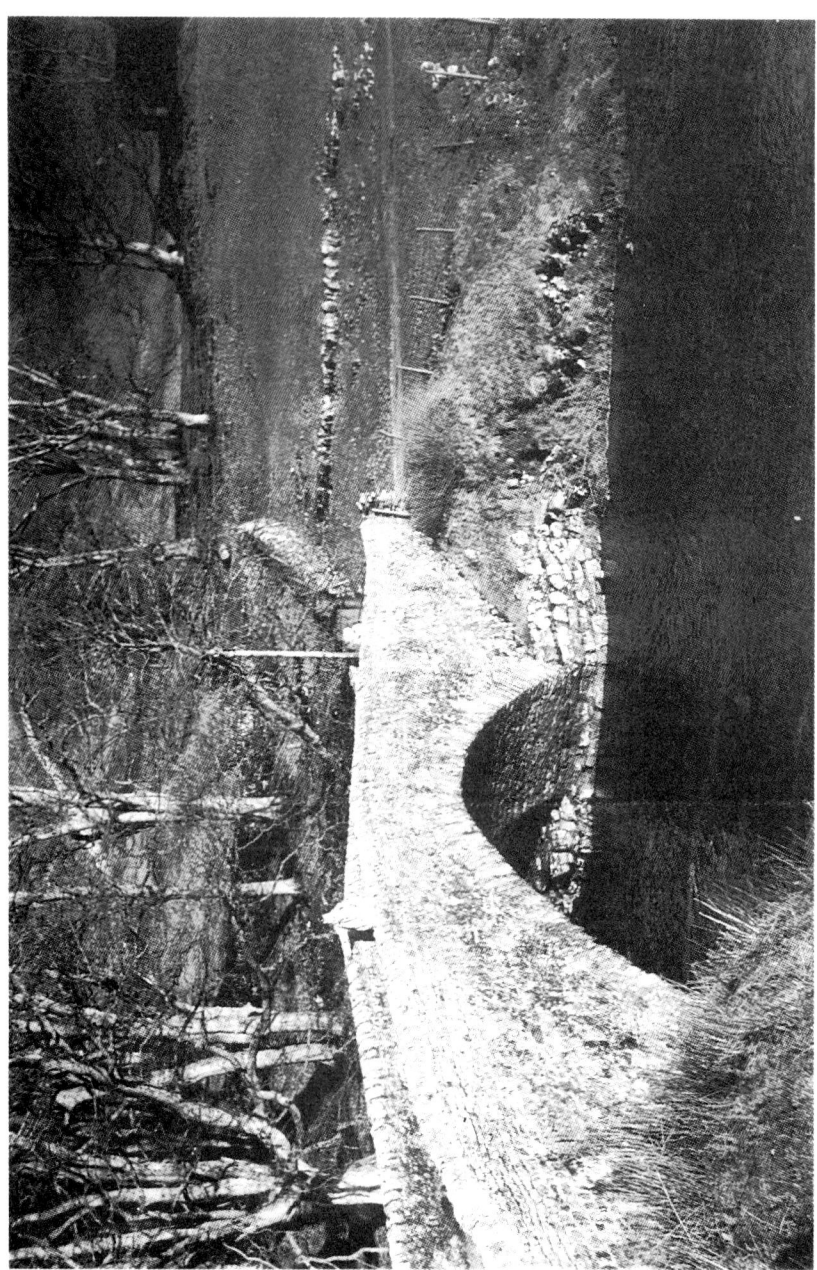

The bridge at Yockenthwaite

LINTON AND ITS SEVEN BRIDGES

The dwellings and the inn surround a spacious green on three sides. A babbling brook which crosses the green from top to bottom is crossed by three bridges – a clapper, a packhorse and a modern one. The clapper bridge, alas, has tarmac on top of the stones and possesses a hand rail which is far from handsome, but the view from it downstream is as lovely as one could wish.

A beautiful old house called White Abbey, once occupied by the novelist Halliwell Sutcliffe, has greensward running down to Threshfield Beck, which joins Linton Beck on its way to the Wharfe river at Linton Mill with its famous falls.

The houses and the inn, The Fountaine, named after Sir Richard Fountaine, are mostly 17th and 18th century. Occupying the west side of the green is a surprisingly large and beautifully-built Almshouse and Hospital, built at the expense of Sir Richard who, with many others, found London streets were actually paved with gold. He was a native of Linton, and in his will of 15th July 1721, he ordered an estate to be purchased, out of which the sum of £26 per annum should be equally divided among six poor men and women of the parish, to be appointed by his trustees and their representatives for ever. The building is said to have cost £1,500. It is thought that Sir John Vanbrugh may well have been the architect, who, on behalf of Sir Richard, planned such a hospital at Enfield, Middlesex; this, however, never got off the ground and it was decided to use the plan to erect it at Linton. It is now looked after by the Fountaine Hospital Trust, and for some years there has been accommodation for four single persons and two couples who have lived or worked in the district. The occupants do not pay rent, but contribute a maintenance fee. In the middle of the building is a chapel, where Evensong is sung each Friday, and Holy Communion is celebrated whenever there is a fifth Sunday in the month. It is usually open to the public for prayer and inspection. A most unusual, indeed unique building of such style for a Dales village.

The village is one of the few which have not grown very much over the past 200 years. The only late 20th century additions to the little streets are the motor cars which appear daily. Even so, Linton is mercifully off the beaten track up and down Wharfedale.

Apart from the seven bridges in the parish, the village can boast of stepping stones over the water near White Abbey. These were formerly in the middle of the village, near the clapper bridge, below the modern bridge. There is also a ford, much of which can be seen just above the packhorse bridge.

The 'Tin' bridge at Linton Falls has been replaced several times over the years, the last time quite recently. It is, of course, a footbridge over which countless visitors have leaned to admire the falls, just about the grandest in the whole of Wharfedale. Unfortunately it hardly matches the falls in the manner of beauty, but we have only to take a few steps to reach Lile Emily's Bridge.

Lile means little in Wharfedale, and no doubt in many other places it is used as a term of endearment or affection. Who then was Lile Emily? She was the daughter of one of the Norton family of Rylston, and at the time of the ill-fated Rising of the North in 1569, the Nortons were in dire trouble. Among those who paid the penalty of execution were Thomas and Christopher Norton. Little Emily, however, was escorted into hiding until the trouble passed, and it was across this little bridge, over the stream formed by the joining of the Linton and Threshfield Becks on their way to the Wharfe, that she went to the cottage of a miller who took care of her. That little stone bridge, so often used by visitors today as a footbridge, has two stone stoops to prevent the free passage of vehicles, however small. It has an attraction of its own. Children love to run over it, and feed the ducks which are ever present, often quite unaware of its name and romantic history. As a reminder of those stirring days, the remains of Norton Tower stand today on the high ground on one's right on approaching Rylston from Skipton.

In the village once again, the road leads us over Linton Beck by means of the 1892 bridge. Leaning over the parapet and looking upstream, this time, the ancient packhorse bridge is only 20 yards away. It has one large main arch which spans the normally shallow water, with more ducks, and one small arch on each side. It is a comely-looking affair, and, in its perfect surroundings, attracts artists and photographers from afar. It is known locally as Redmayne's Bridge, because it was rebuilt at the expense of Mrs Elizabeth Redmayne c 1690, and originally built at least 100 years before that. Mrs Redmayne, who died in 1718, was a native of Linton, and a brass memorial plate to her can be seen in Linton church, which is a delightful hoary and steadfast reminder of how Christianity has stood the test of time.

The old route from Skipton via Lauradale Lane crossed the beck in Linton and joined the Burnsall-Threshfield road. From there it descended towards Lile Emily's Bridge, but, just before doing so, turned left, passing over yet another old bridge of stone, and then alongside the Old Grammar School. Soon after that, it turned right and passed over Linton's seventh bridge, known nowadays as Grassington Bridge. This old route is said to have crossed the Wharfe by 'Linton brig of stone over Wharfe fluv.' From there it follows the east side of the valley to Conistone and beyond.

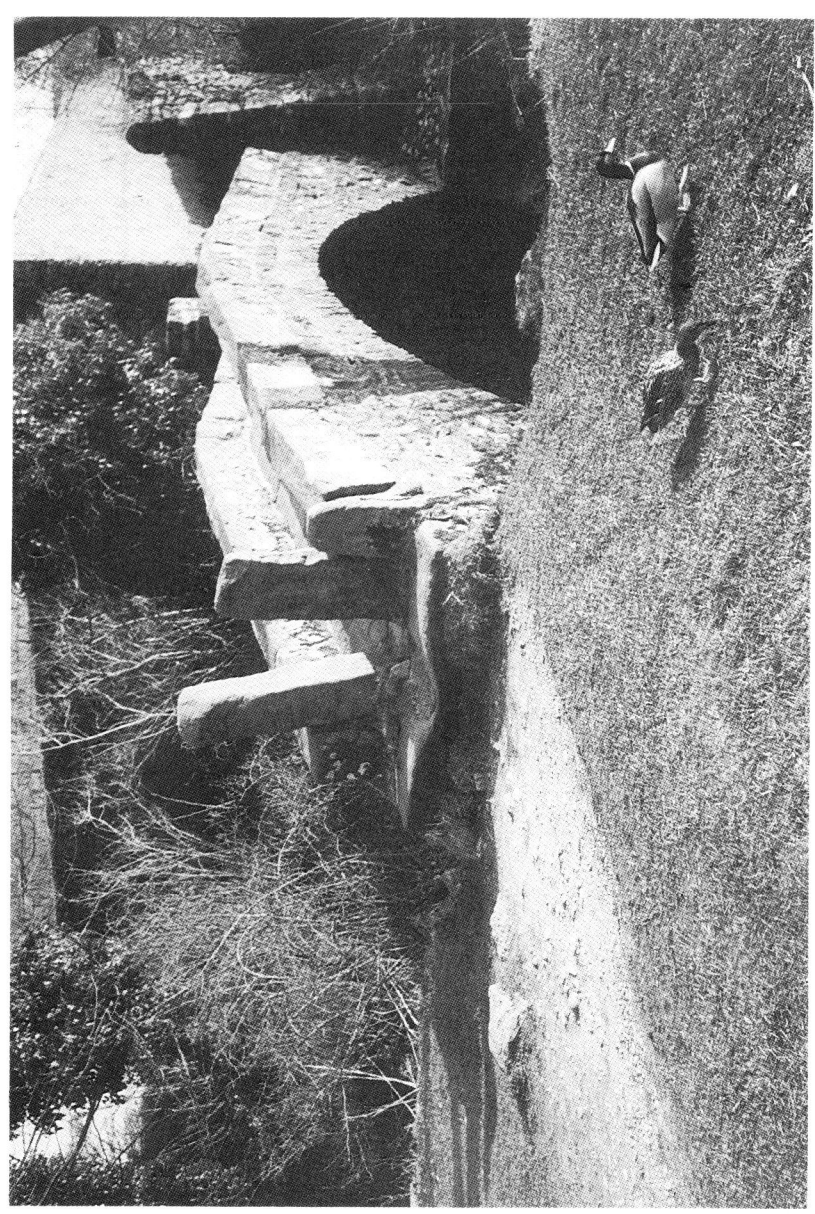

Lile Emily's Bridge in Linton

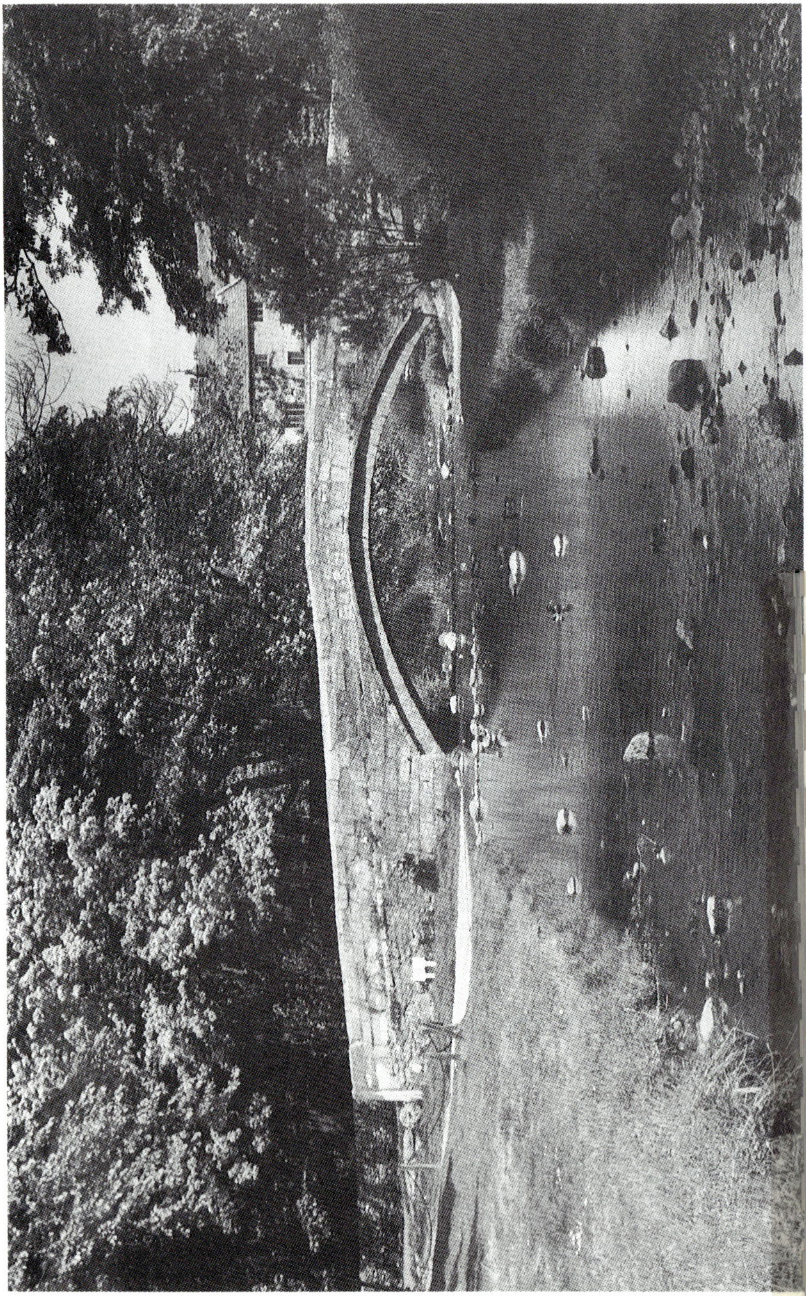

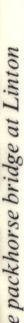

The packhorse bridge at Linton

Actually, only the northern end of the bridge is in Grassington.

Grassington Bridge replaced in 1603 a derelict wooden structure, and is the oldest existing bridge in Upper Wharfedale. It was originally a hump-backed affair, repaired in 1661 and widened in 1783, and eventually raised to its present level at each end, thus avoiding the hump in the middle. In 1984, it was widened yet again on the upstream side. Under the four segmental arches, the stages of building can be seen quite easily, as the segment of the downstream portion does not quite coincide with that of the upstream arch. Furthermore, the outline of the former hump-back is plainly seen, along with the masonry which filled in the space left by raising the carriageway at each end.

The whole has an appeal, especially the view from downstream, and it is not surprising that it is the subject of so many photographs and paintings.

If the builders of 1603 were alive today, they would be justly proud of their handiwork. While so many Wharfedale bridges were turned over during the great flood of 1673, Grassington Bridge remained firm, so that it looks as if the repairs to an already sturdy bridge were well and truly tested, and, maybe, timely.

BARDEN BRIDGE

Approaching Barden Tower from the riverside path from Appletreewick, the first thing one sees is a graceful stone bridge of three segmental arches, with massive pointed cutwaters which provide niches in the parapets. It is a well-used bridge, but decidedly hump-backed. One-way traffic is the order of the day, as there is only about 10 feet between the parapets.

A bridge existed in the 14th century, and probably before that. Some £300 was spent, it is said, in 1659, but only 14 years later the bridge was washed away in the great inundation of water of 1673. However, by 1676 it was completely rebuilt, as per the tablet to be seen on the parapet approach wall:

> THIS BRIDGE WAS
> REPAYRED AT THE
> CHARGE OF THE
> WHOLE WEST RIDING
> 1676

Major repairs were made and new parapets placed in 1856, and again in 1955, following successions of flood damage. It is gratifying to see that the bridge today is no wider than it was 300 or more years ago. Traffic bent on speed to reach Burnsall, Linton, Grassington and beyond have no need to use the bridge, because the main road up the dale, after passing Barden Tower, goes straight on, thus avoiding the steep and twisting descent to the river. It is most pleasant to stand in one of the niches and contemplate the romantic history with which this area is so closely associated, while watching the clear waters of the Wharfe with their everlasting flow waiting for no man.

Readers will, no doubt, have realized that Leland's opinion of the state of bridges in Upper Airedale and Upper Wharfedale has not been given. The fact is that he had no remarks to make. For some unknown reason, he never gave the area a visit, but this is what he said:

> "Ribil riseth in Ribilsdale above Sally Abbey and so to Sawley. A IILI miles above Sawley it reseyvith Calder that cummitt by Walley and after reseyvith another Cawllid Oder. Bishopdale lyeth joyinynge to the quarters of Craven. Cover River riseth, as I here say, in Cravenside, enr Skale Park. Richmondshire lieth hard on the borders of Cravenland. Craven lyeth south-weste from Richmondshire."

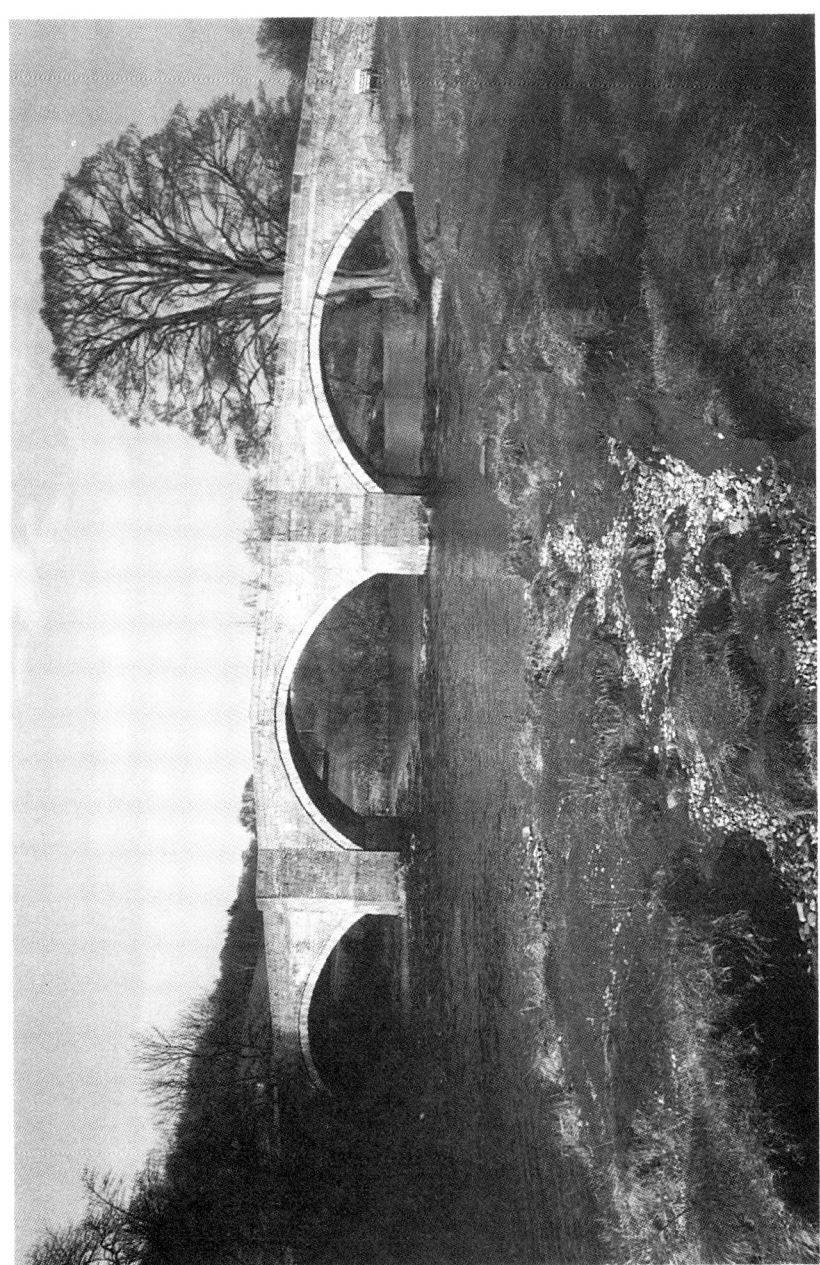

Barden Bridge

The bridge is said to have been crossed by young William Craven, a farmer's son on the start of his journey, in the charge of a carrier, to London. In due course, he became apprenticed to a mercer and his diligence and thrift were rewarded eventually by success and wealth. In 1611 he became Lord Mayor of London. He was knighted, and endowed Burnsall Grammar School. He also bore the cost of restoring the church and rebuilding the bridge at Burnsall, among many other needs of the day.

The history of Barden Tower and bridge is bound up with the Clifford family dating back to the 11th century. John, Lord Clifford, or Blackfaced (Butcher) Clifford, who brutally killed the young Earl of Rutland in cold blood during the Battle of Wakefield, was so hated by the Yorkists that revenge was in the minds of the latter. However, a year later, the Butcher met his death through a stray arrow on the eve of the Battle of Towton. The Yorkists were, of course, victorious here and the Butcher's son, Henry, Lord Clifford, only a boy, was taken secretly from Skipton to Threlkeld in Cumbria, as it was feared that he would still be the victim of revenge. He led the life of a shepherd for something like 20 years, until the Houses of York and Lancaster were joined by marriage. Warlike strife ceased, and the young Clifford, who became known as the Shepherd Lord, returned home to the hunting lodge at Barden. He enlarged it into what is now known as Barden Tower in 1485. By 1589, however, the Tower became sadly neglected, and, in the years following, fell into ruin. The indefatigable Lady Anne Clifford had the place restored when she married the Earl of Dorset. He died in 1624, and 1630 in she married the Earl of Pembroke. The restoration included the chapel which had been founded by the Shepherd Lord.

The whole appears to have remained intact until at least 1774, after which it fell into ruin once again, though it now forms a picturesque scene, well-maintained and popular with visitors. In the stonework of the Tower is a fresh-looking tablet which elaborates the story for visitors, in quaint lettering:

THIS BARDEN TOWER WAS REPAYRED
BY THE LADIE ANNE CLIFFORD COVNTE
SSE DOWAGER OF PEMBROKE DORSETT
AND MONTGEMERY BARONESSE CLIFFORD
WESTMERLAND AND VESEIE LADY OF THE
HONOR OF SKIPTON IN CRAVEN AND HIGH
SHERIFESSE BY INHERITANCE OF THE
COVNTIE OF WESTMERLAND IN THE YEARES

1658 AND 1659 AFTER ITT HAD LAYNE
RVINOVS EVER SINCE ABOVT 1589 WHEN
HER MOTHER THEN LAY IN ITT AND WAS
GREATE WITH CHILD WITH HER TILL
NOWE THAT ITT WAS REPAYRD BY
THE SAYD LADY. 1ST CHAP 58 VER 1
GODS NAME BE PRAISED

BOLTON BRIDGE

As mentioned in the chapter on Kildwick, the Augustinian Canons founded a priory at Embsay, but found it was not to their liking and moved to Bolton, where they remained until 1539. Fortunately, the King allowed the nave to remain as a parish church.

Bolton Bridge, originally 12th century, had a chapel, like Wakefield and Rotherham, for the benefit of travellers who wished to receive God's Blessing for the remainder of their journey. The bridge was rebuilt of wood by the Canons in 1313/14 at a cost of £13:6:8d and paid for by the prior's mother, Eve of Laund, the hamlet to the north of the present wooden bridge which crosses the river near the Cavendish Pavilion.

Ferryhouse, occupied for many years by Mr Donald Wood, Church-warden Emeritus, stands at the west end of the bridge. It is notable for a wooden beam on which are carved and painted in red the words:

THOW YAT PASSYS BY YES WAY
ONE AVE MARIA HERE YOU SAY

Shenstone, the poet, inspired by the Priory and its lovely environment, wrote:

"While through the land the musing pilgrim sees a brighter tract of brighter green and in the midst appears a mouldering wall with ivy crowned, or gothic turret, pride of ancient days".

Pilgrims would surely cross the bridge* where the valley suddenly widens, and the Wharfe flows through fertile meadows and pastures after a turbulent passage through Bolton Woods.

According to traditions, Prince Rupert encamped here on his way to historic Marston Moor in July 1644.

It was not so long after this that the bridge was washed away, like so many others in the dale, in the great flood of 1673, but it was soon replaced, owing to its importance as the Lancester to York road crossed the Wharfe here. A short distance up the road on the left is the remarkable Beamsley Hospital, entry to which is gained through an ancient arch to a quite unusual circular building. It was founded towards the end of the 16th century, and some 60 years later, Lady Anne Clifford provided additional amenities and improvements. It will be recollected that this lady's initials (in colour) appear as A P 1655 on two windows in Skipton Parish Church,

which she restored in many ways in 1655. On two other windows the letter P 1655 appears. She left her mark on more places than that!
*Note: About to be bypassed.

ILKLEY AND ITS BRIDGE

Ilkley is certainly famous for its moor if not its bridge. However, that very moor displays visible evidence of prehistoric man, whose rock carvings of all descriptions are in abundance. Cup and Ring stones are found over a very wide area. The most notable carved stone, near the edge of the moor overlooking Ilkley, is the Swastika Stone, unique in this country. The only other identical one known is at Tossene in Sweden.

Ilkley was granted a market way back in the 13th century, but this appears to have lapsed very many years ago. It was an important Roman station, however, and the stone remains of the fort are still to be seen to this day. The parish church of All Saints stands on part of the site and dates from AD 1074. On the site to the west of the church stands the attractive Manor House museum, which, with the church, is a great storehouse of history. Saxon crosses are to be seen in the church itself.

In early Victorian times, the town suddenly became famous for its Hydropathic Establishments, sadly out of date now, but Iklkey is always thronged with visitors on 'The Grove' and the riverside between the old and new bridges, as well as on the moor, especially near the Cow and Calf rocks.

Our route is down Brook Street as far as the new bridge, then upstream on either side of the river Wharfe to the Old Bridge. The latter is a traditional three-arched crossing of stone. The two outer arches each have a span of something like 30ft, but the central arch has a span of 50ft and as a consequence rises much higher than the other two. This in turn causes quite a hump in the middle. It dates from 1678, but years before that the Romans, as one might expect, had a crossing hereabouts. If one takes into account the fact that most of their fort of Olicana stood west of New Brook Street, then the Roman crossing would be most likely a little downstream from the present Old Bridge. In fact, there are many large stones on or near the banks of the river which the romantically-inclined historian could label as being of Roman origin.

It is said that the Roman 'executive' Clodius Fronto was misled by the apparently shallowness of the water and slipped on the pebble bed, getting a thorough wetting. As Olicana was on the main Roman military way from Manchester to Aldborough, and on the road from York to Ribchester, a bridge would surely have superceded a ford if Clodius Fronto had had anything to do with it!

There was certainly a bridge in Leland's time, circa 1530, but is seems to have been a source of trouble from 1638 (when it was partly rebuilt) to 1670. Those 32 years saw much expense being authorized at various

Sessions. This was all to no avail, because in 1673 continual very heavy rain caused a flood of such volume that Ilkley Bridge, like so many others in Wharfedale, was overturned.

Five years later, the present bridge was constructed and has stood the test of time and weather, apart from odd repairs, in spite of floods in 1866, 1936 and 1966.

By the 1880s, the traffic had become such that the dear old bridge was considered inadequate, especially on account of it having such a high pitch. Horse-drawn vehicles would suddenly come face to face at the highest point, and the harangueing between the drivers in a situation like that needs no imagination.

In 1884, moves were made to widen it, but these gave way to a feeling that another bridge should be built much further downstream. However, it was not until 1904 that a new metal bridge was constructed at the bottom of Brook Street, and formally opened in 1906. It was many years after that before the old bridge was finally closed to all traffic except pedestrians. Now it is there to lean over, without let or hindrance, to be fascinated with the water's various moods. Incidentally, the modern Dales Way, traversed by many walkers, starts at the south end.

Let us hope that at least some of the work of late 20th century artists will be available for future generations to admire in, say, AD 2500 and realize what the bridge looked like today.

In the Domesday Book, ILCLIEVE was regarded as part of the great Manor of Otley, our next port of call.

OTLEY

As one approaches Otley from, say, Bradford, a large sign on the left indicates that the visitor is about to enter an historic market town. How true! It was an ancient Saxon Borough, and the story of its equally ancient parish church of All Saints, with its lovely peal of bells, almost warrants a book to itself.

The importance of Otley, even at the time of the Conquest, cannot be gainsaid. Its Manor covered nearly 30,000 acres on both sides of the river Wharfe. It had a market granted in 1222, and records show that in 1378, 43 married couples and 25 single persons paid Poll Tax. In the Civil War, the parish of Otley provided no less a personage than Sir Thomas Fairfax of Denton Hall (near Otley) as leader.

Otley was half-way between Knaresborough and Skipton (both garrison towns), and it is reliably reported that when Cromwell led his army in Yorkshire, he camped the night in Otley and some of his soldiers drank dry the old inn (Black Bull) in the market place.

The Free Grammar School was founded about 1602 in a one-storey building, and Thomas Fairfax was one of the trustees. A beautifully-built edifice succeeded it on the north side of manor Square. Alas, the school was subsequently closed owing to lack of sufficient endowment. It is now a glass and china shop, and the school (Prince Henry's) is at present across the river.

How could a town of such history and romance – far too many great events to enumerate here – exist without a great bridge across the river? To reach the ancient bridge, one passes through Manor Square to Clapgate and then down Northgate (now called Bridge Street), passing the Old Smithy (now a doctors' surgery). Note the old iron ring still fixed to the side of the one-time doorway. Lower down is the office of the oldest agricultural show in England – The Wharfedale Agricultural Society. A one-time competitor at the show was a famous Irish-born ox, which had been reared in Yorkshire. It weighed 254 stones and was said to be the biggest in the world – important enough to have its head preserved and kept in York Castle Museum. To complete the picture, at the lower end of the street stood, until 1928, the old Toll Bar House, a relic of the turnpike days.

Now we reach the bridge, and on the left is the entrance to a pleasant stretch of greensward and riverside path open to the public.

John Leland, who was given the title of Royal Antiquary by Henry VIII, visited Otley on his travels and according to him, Otley Bridge was a stone structure before the Reformation, but there was most certainly a bridge at the time of the Conquest. It could have been of wood or stone and wood and in the twelfth century the lepers of the then Otley Hospital in Westgate had to keep it in repair. This procedure did not last very long, however, for Archbishop Gray in 1226 granted an indulgence of thirteen days to those who would contribute to the building of a new bridge. The Archbishop, aided by private benefactors, maintained the bridge for some 40 years, until the first act of Parliament was passed for the repair and maintenance of roads and bridges of public utility.

In 1673, the bridge was swept away, along with several others higher up the dale, in the worst flood waters on record. Thereafter, the present bridge of seven segmental arches (across the widest part of the Wharfe hereabouts) was built, and widened on the west side in 1776 following storm damage in 1774. In more recent years, a projecting footway has been erected on the east side, thus allowing the main carriageway to be vehicular. There have been several serious floods since the last rebuilding took place, but the bridge has withstood them all. It spans a total of 80 yards with very little rise in height towards the middle. A remarkable piece of workmanship, and what a vast and varied amount of traffic it has carried, from cattle, travelling circuses and theatres, as well as small armies, cattle trucks and the ubiquitous motor car.

The river Wharfe has a large and important tributary – the Washburn – which, before it enters the Wharfe, fills no less than four reservoirs. It rises in the hills and allotments to the north-west of the drowned village of West End. Washburn Head is on the eastern boundary of the Yorkshire Dales National Park, and the Washburn enters the Wharfe a few miles east of Otley, but the bridges which span it are not of very special interest, except one which lies between Swinsty Reservoir and Lindley Reservoir.

Deep down well-wooded slopes, very steep, stands Dob Park packhorse bridge, its noble arch of stone standing well above the water. It appears to be segmental, and the parapet has a very obtuse-angled high point. The approach 'roads' on both sides are very steep, and that from the south, particularly, cannot be described as a motor road! Nevertheless its attractions are manifold, and the walker is well-rewarded from whichever side of the valley he approaches it. The bridge is said to date from the 16th century, and the ancient parish of Fewston was responsible for its upkeep. It was rebuilt in 1738 at a cost of £50.

At low water, the remains of a ford, well-paved, can be seen and the crossing suggests a one-time packhorse route from Otley over the tops into the Nidd valley.

WETHERBY

About halfway between London and Edinburgh, Wetherby is situated on the north bank of the Wharfe, which flows in the narrow gorge in the magnesian limestone belt like the Nidd at Knaresborough.

The original bridge is said to date back to the 11th century and was eleven feet wide, but the present one was rebuilt and widened in 1824, and the stones of the original are incorporated in it. Furthermore, those stones are said to be from the ruins of a castle which stood on the high north bank – Castle Garth. The latter was probably built by the Percy family, who were owners of the land at Wetherby as well as many parts of Wharfedale. The Castle was, for a short time, a possession of the Knights Templar, who were, as previously mentioned, established at Ribston. However, the years 1312/3 saw the beginning of the end of the Templars as such, and coincidentally with this, the bridge was in need of repair. In 1315, repairs were undertaken by the widow of Henry de Perci. Previous to this, one of the Vavasour family put up the sum of £1 towards repair!

In addition to the bridge, the old ford still existed, and to evade toll some travellers took advantage of this. They got off scot-free until Wetherby men decided, after the dodgers had had their way for some twelve months, to charge a toll whichever way the travellers chose to make the crossing.

It is on record that, during the Civil Wars, Sir Thomas Fairfax defended Wetherby and its bridge in 1642.

Wetherby, being on the Great North Road, would witness the drovers who came from Scotland with great herds of cattle. Some of the cattle on their way south would be attended to by the village blacksmith and fitted with shoes to ease their journey.

The town was, of course, an important coaching station, and if there was a shortage of accommodation, it was only a short step to Walshford, and vice-versa.

Let us have a close look at the bridge as it stands today. It is a fine structure of six almost semi-circular arches, very high above the river. Apart from those at Ferrybridge and Castleford, it is regarded as the finest in Yorkshire. The upstream side appears to be the older and has five large cutwaters, but on the downstream side they are small and not very high. In spite of the fact that the modern A1 by-passes the town, the old bridge is busy, and reminiscent, in a different way perhaps, of the days when the Knights Templar held a market at Wetherby following their acquisition of land there, having been transferred from Walshford.

TADCASTER

The Calcaria of Roman Times!

Here the Wharfe cuts its way through the widest gap in the limestone belt. Limestone burning has taken place here for as far back as memory takes us. No doubt, this is why the Romans thought fit to give the name they did. Ainsty, the ancient County of York City, was a well-cultivated, well-wooded and well-watered area west of York, with Tadcaster the chief town.

At this point, we might well mention how Leland came to embark on his "Itinerary", especially the Yorkshire portion. King Henry VIII, in the 25th year of his reign, gave a "moste gratius commission" to him to "peruse and diligently to serche all the Libraries of Monasteries and Collegies of this – Reaulme . . as of this Province might be brought out of deadely darkness to lyvely lighte". By virtue of this commission, Leland traversed the greater portion of England and Wales. The result of these travels was his celebrated "Itinerary" "which was geven of him as a Newe Yeare's Gyfte to King Henry the VIII in the XXXVII Yeare of his Raygne".

As regards Tadcaster, Leland said, "Tadcaster standeth on the hither ripe of Wharf river, and is a good thoroughfare. The bridge over Wharf hath eight fair arches of stone. Some say that it was last made of the ruins of the old castle. A mighty great gill, dykes and garth of the castle on Wharf may yet be seen a little above the bridge. It seemeth by the plot that it was a right stately thing".

Today, the bridge retains its ancient charm, though obviously altered since Leland's time, as only five semi-circular arches are now visible. The castle, which once stood upstream from the bridge and church of St Mary's, is gone except for the scant remains of motte and bailey. As Leland suggests, the castle stones were used to build and indeed re-build the bridge, which is very attractive viewed from either up or down stream, even though widened in the 19th century. It displays small decorations, and forms an attractive picture viewed from downstream with the church tower in the background. The older part of the structure is upstream, and its rounded cutwaters of old grey stone add to its charm, whilst the cutwaters on the downstream side are pointed.

Tadcaster was also the scene of battle. Sir Thomas Fairfax and his Parliamentarians fought in its very streets against the Earl of Newcastle in 1642.

We cannot take leave of Tadcaster without referring to its brewing industry, which has been sustained for over 600 years, and also its corn mills:

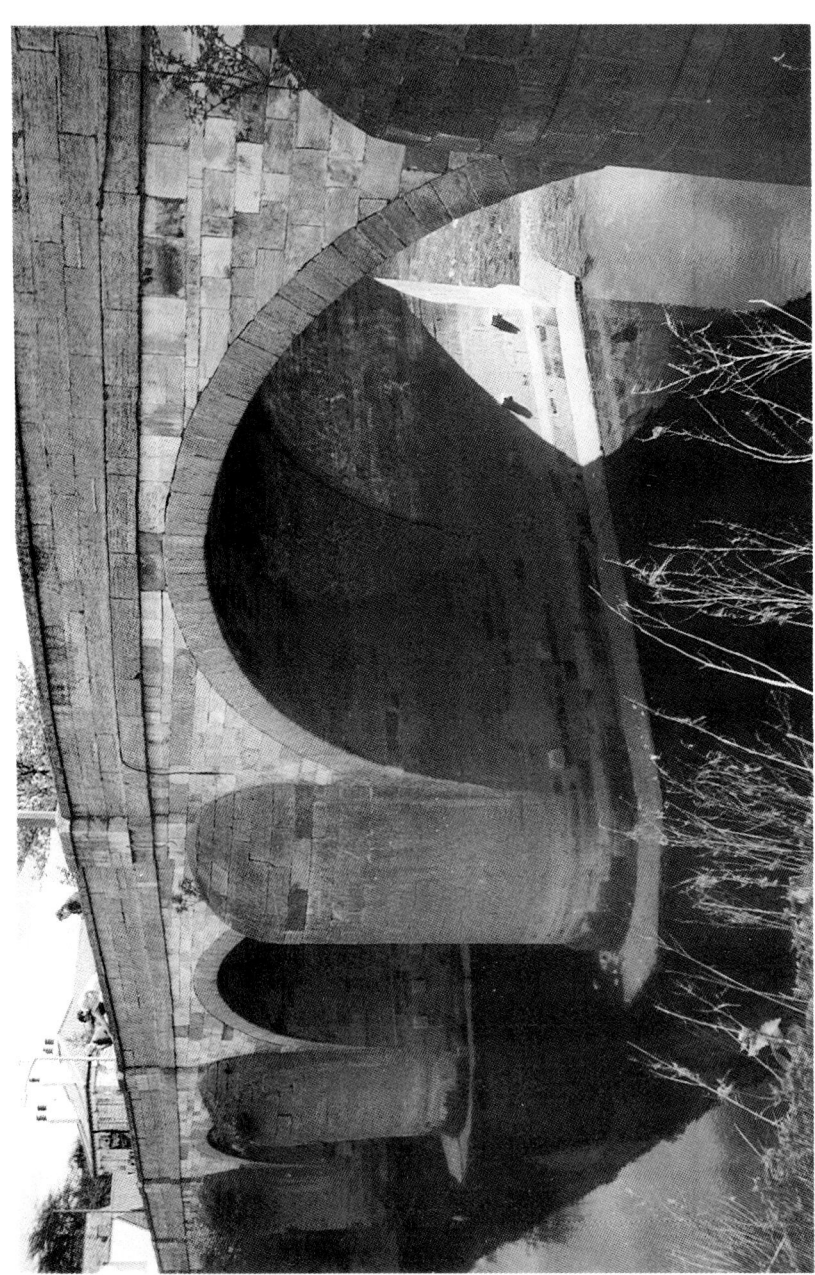

Tadcaster Bridge from upstream

Of all the landward towns in that great haughty shire,
Old Tadcaster on Wharfe the highest may aspire;
To her belongs a grace that ever will avail
In her right and honest meal, and better still, her ale;
For there the sovereign draught its power may never fear,
As it can elsewhere find no rival, and no peer.

CAWOOD

Wharfedale, particularly the part between Ilkley and Kettlewell, and, to a lesser extent, Buckden and Hubberholme, is, of course, well known to its many visitors. Comparatively few seem to know where the river Wharfe ends its long journey and joins the Ouse.

We cannot let this lovely river disappear into the Ouse without having a look at the little town of Cawood, which stands on the Ouse, even though it has no bridge of the kind we have so far visited. The river is tidal here, and a ferry existed from time immemorial until 1872, when a steel bridge was built. Today a lofty tower stands in the middle and barriers drop down when the bridge is about to swing open for the passage of river traffic. Just round the bend upstream, the Wharfe pours its waters into the Ouse.

Long before 1872, the trade route between the Scandinavian countries and Ireland came via the Humber, the Ouse and Cawood. Wouldn't those traders just have loved the Aire and Calder and Leeds and Liverpool Canals? Years later the Romans used the ford at Cawood on their journey from Castleford to York. Athelstan, the first King of all England, gave the manors of Cawood and Sherburn to Wulfstan, Archbishop of York, to commemorate his victory over the Scots and Danes in the 10th century. The Normans strengthened Cawood, and from then on it became the seat of the Archbishops of York and a regular second home for royalty. The castle extended right to the river bank, but the gatehouse was entered from the side now remote from the present road. Among the many royal visitors was Edward I, with his second wife, Margaret, who gave birth to the first Duke of Norfolk at Brotherton near Ferrybridge in 1300.

Dick Turpin and his horse, the famous Black Bess, crossed the river at Cawood when riding from London to York.

The white stone gatehouse is all that remains of the original castle; it is very attractive and one can stay there on a self-catering holiday. Above the massive oak doors of the former entrance there are a living room and kitchen; above those a bedroom and bathroom. The property is owned by the Landmark Trust.

For a brief history lesson about the enthronement of George Neville as Archbishop of York, one might well visit the Ferry Inn. There, on a large plaque, is the astounding menu of the Great Feast to celebrate his coming enthronement. On 15th January 1466 (St Maurice's Day), Cawood Castle saw the greatest feast ever recorded. It is said that over 8,000 people gathered there from miles around, and many came from York to participate in the event, which lasted several days. More than 1000 were employed to cook and serve the food, seven courses in all. Included in the menu were 500 stags, bucks and roes, 1000 muttons, 2000 geese, 4000 pasties of venison, 3000 baked custards (cold) and 2000 hot custards, 300 tuns of ale and 100 tuns of wine.

George Neville's effort only enhanced his reputation for a short time, and after seven years he was stripped of everything and sent to prison in France, having incurred the King's displeasure.

Cardinal Wolsey, who, after being made Chancellor of England by Henry VIII, fell out of favour with the King (agreed with him over his divorce of Katherine of Aragon, but agreed also with the Pope's opinion) was sent to Cawood in 1530. After settling in at Cawood, three weeks before his actual enthronement as Archbishop of York, Wolsey was arrested by the Earl of Northumberland on a charge of high treason. The rest of the sad story of Wolsey we all know.

The year 1646 saw the end of Cawood staging the splendour of Royalty and Archbishops. The castle was voted by the House of Commons as redundant. Much of the stone was removed and used to build the entrance of Bishopthorpe, the Archbishops' present palace at York.

Cawood is the point where the old Bishop's Dyke joins the Ouse. The dyke was built to run from Sherburn to the town, and its waters provided power for corn mills. At one time, Huddlestone Quarry near Sherburn sent limestone via the dyke to Cawood, and thence to the Ouse to York, for building purposes, especially for repairing, and indeed building, some of the Minster.

And so Cawood, proud of its long history and regarded as the Windsor of the North, stands serenely beside the Ouse – so many people quite unaware of its existence, let alone its momentous history; a town largely dependent on river traffic and trade, consequently without much wheeled traffic in the side streets, which are very narrow and consist of quaint little alleyways.

KILDWICK

Having left behind us the romantic beginnings of the Aire and historic Skipton, we are now well and truly in the Aire Gap and its river, which bears much of the brunt of the Industrial Revolution. From now on it seems fated to have modern industry along its banks, as well as that of the past. We must admit, however, that industry created much of the wealth which made our country great. Its very presence in the Aire Gap through the Pennines contributed to the importance of the commercial and trade route from West Yorkshire to East Lancashire.

Whilst many of the rural Yorkshire Dales and the river Derwent had their own industries such as lead mining, cotton and flax as well as corn mills, they largely escaped the effects of the Industrial Revolution. Airedale, Calderdale, the Don valley and their tributaries can rival the others in stirring events in the history of England. Kildwick in the Aire valley, in spite of its position between Keighley and Skipton, and the fact that the Leeds and Liverpool Canal divides it, for the most part, from its close neighbour. Farnhill, still retains its ancient features without modern additions. Even the canal presents one of its most picturesque sections here, and passes over the road which joins the two villages.

Let us have a close look at the old stone bridge as it crosses the Aire. Until the opening, during the last decade, of the western part of the Aire Valley trunk road, Kildwick was on the main road from Keighley to Kendal, and, of course, its bridge gave good passage over the river. Some two hundred years before this, the Keighley to Kendal turnpike passed this way; the turnpike trust was formed in 1753, and by 1780 the turnpike was in full swing. The bridge's oldest portion is found on the upstream side and the arches are well groyned; the widening took place in 1780 on the downstream side and seems to be consistent with the opening up of the turnpike. A peep under the arches reveals the 'new', part which nearly doubles the original width. In this connection, it is interesting to note that, some 130 years ago, Dr Whitaker, in his 'History of Craven', states:

> "the bridge at Kildwick is a monument to the well-judged liberality of the canons of Bolton, by whom it was built in the Reign of Edward II (It has been widened and its ancient appearance destroyed)."

Many old bridges have one or more arches which are pointed, the rest being rounded. Kildwick has two of each on the upstream side, but downstream all four are rounded, so one can perhaps appreciate Dr Whitaker's remarks!

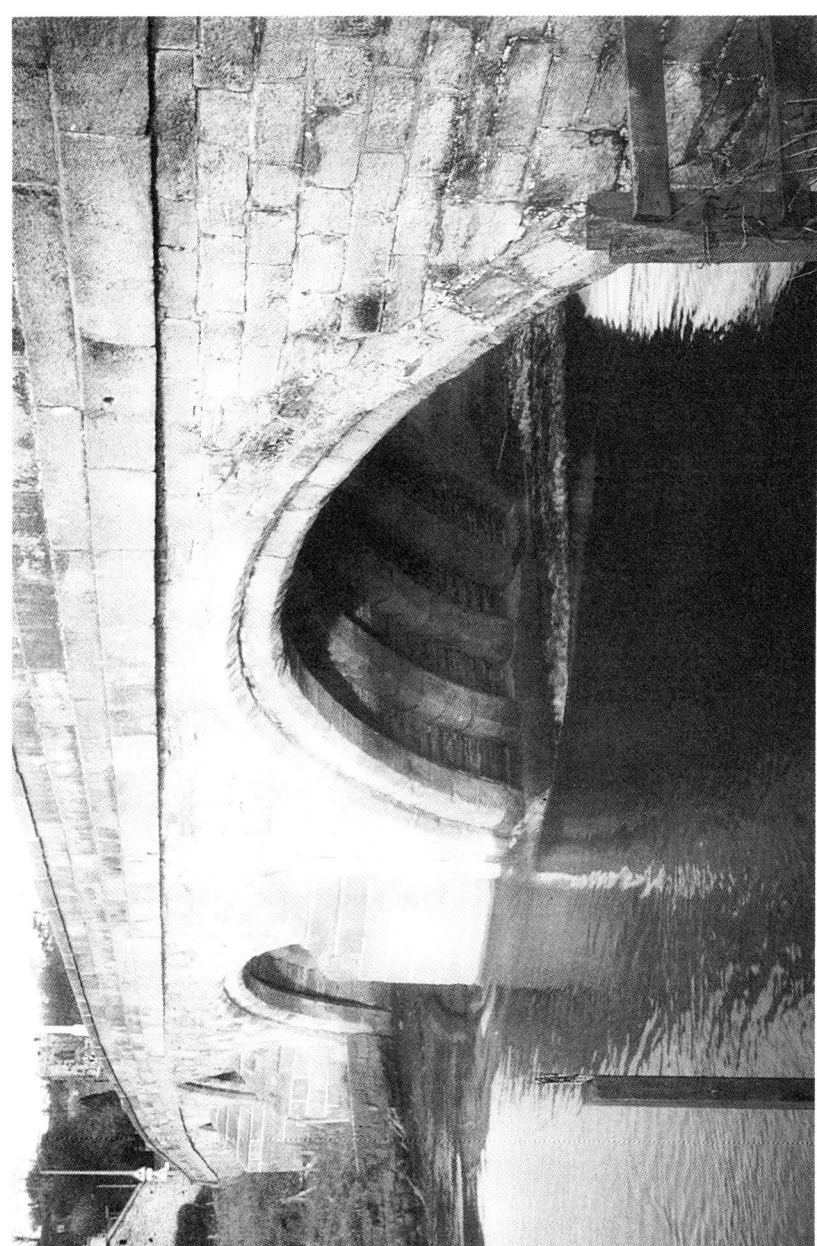

Kildwick Bridge

It seems that over the centuries the river has brought down a considerable amount of silt and pebbles, which have built up against the northern end of the bridge, resulting in a large, green, but rather wet, field. As a result, the river normally flows through the two rounded arches only.

According to records at Bolton Abbey (Priory), the bridge was built c 1305 at a cost of £21:12:9d! The Manor of Kildwick came under the jurisdiction of the then priors and the bridge was built to serve both the Priory and Kildwick church, and ever since has been an important crossing.

Now the dear old bridge has stood little change for the past two hundred years, and for nearly five hundred years before that in its narrow state; the traffic has abated, and peace (almost) is the order of the day whilst unending heavy (and light) traffic thunders over its nearby modern counterpart a little upstream.

Here we have once again, the Bridge, the Church and the Inn forming a trio. Crossing the bridge from the south, one's immediate view is of the inn – the White Lion – and the church tower with its attractive clock face. The hostelry was always associated with the church and its affairs.

If the name of the village is anything to go by, it must go back to the Norse invasion of Yorkshire in pre-conquest times: childe (a well or spring) and uuic (a place in which to dwell). Kildwick (Childeuuic) appears in the Domesday Book of 1086, and in c 1100 it, along with much of the Craven district, passed to Robert de Romille, whose daughter, Cecilia, founded a priory at Embsay which was moved some 50 years later to Bolton, at that delightful bend in the river Wharfe over the hill to the north. For something like four hundred years, the Manor seems to have pursued the even tenor of its way until Henry VIII thought otherwise. Thereafter it came into the possession of two clothiers, a Robert Wilkinson of Bradford and Thomas Drake of Halifax, who, according to Dr Whitaker, sold it to a John Garforth (one of the great family of Garforth who lived at Steeton Hall for several hundred years), who in turn sold it to Henry Currer. The Currers were Lords of the Manor from c 1600 for over 150 years. Their home was Kildwick Hall, high above the village.

The old vicarage, originally built prior to the Civil War, is reached from the church by means of a picturesque bridge over the canal, and through an archway with a stone cross inset at the head. Thereafter, the way up is by a very steep flagged path at the side of a stream.

The church itself, the Lang Kirk of Craven, certainly lives up to its name, having been lengthened in the 16th century. Its total length is approximately 145 feet. It is the largest in the Craven Deanery, and one of the largest in Yorkshire. Inside the church, one is immediately struck by its beauty as well as its size. It is thought that the first church here was in existence as far back as AD 940; in any case, a stone church was erected in the 12th century. A 26-page booklet by Mr Alec Wood, 'History and Description of the Church of St Andrew, Kildwick in Craven', is a rare companion to have in one's possession whilst exploring Kildwick, its church, its bridge, its ancient hostelry and many other fascinating places of interest.

Across the 18th century canal is the unique village of Farnhill, consisting mainly of a level street parallel with the canal, with a number of quaint and very steep streets leading up from it. The village store and post office, with its great variety of goods, faces the canal and quaint houses on the Kildwick side. Mallards and their mates complete the picture. An extraordinary place, little Farnhill, of whose existence tens of thousands of motorists tearing along the new trunk road are quite unaware. Mounting one of those steep streets, which get steeper as one climbs, we find that pleasant modern houses put in an appearance right up the old high road. Turn to the right and see Kildwick Hall; turn to left, and shortly beyond the village Farnhill Manor House appears ahead on a rounded and wooded knoll.

Back to Kildwick again, we go through the churchyard, past the church – a veritable treasure house – to the internal car park, where we see a quite unique tombstone to the memory of John Laycock, organ builder. The carefully carved stone takes the form of a church organ, complete with pipes and design, of the first organ built by him. In the street below, near the war memorial, are the stone stocks, and opposite the White Lion are double mounting steps and a sundial dated 1668.

At the bridge once more, and standing in that wet and soggy field, we cannot fail to admire the skill and dedication of the builders. Every stone needed to be shaped by hand with great care, and the foundations laid in the river without modern equipment, so many hundreds of years ago. One wonders whether or not the builders stood back and admired their handiwork. What a wonderful legacy they have left us, especially the beauty of it all.

DOWN THE AIRE VALLEY TO CASTLEFORD AND FERRYBRIDGE

Our next bridge of special note is at Bingley, a little town with a long and eventful history. We must content ourselves with its bridge, however, and to see it, we turn sharply down to the right after passing the ancient church of All Saints. It is known as Ireland Bridge and dates back to 1685, the year the previous wooden structure was dismantled. Packhorses with their tinkling bells were frequent users of it as it was an important crossing of the Aire – there was no other crossing at one time until Apperley Bridge was reached many miles down river.

Ireland Bridge? It seems that because the south and north sides of the river belonged to different manors and owners, and as a sizeable stretch of water separated them, some likened the situation to England and Ireland! Likely story or not, the name remains. Before those days, the Romans built a road from Luddenden (Calderdale) to Ilkley (Wharfedale) and it passed this way.

Across the bridge, a path leads to Beckfoot Bridge. It is very attractive, and crosses Harden Beck just before the latter joins the Aire. It is, of course, a footbridge only, built of stone about 1723. With such a high arch, the handrailings are essential, but do not seem to detract from its appearance, judging by the number of artists and photographers who frequently visit it. Instead of crossing the bridge which leads to Myrtle Park, we follow a narrow lane high up on the southern bank of the Aire and emerge at Cottingley Bridge. This was built of stone in 1779/80, and is a pleasing and well-built structure of four arches. It carries an enormous amount of heavy traffic, hardly contemplated some 200 years ago, which says a great deal for the skill and devotion to the work of the builder, a Thomas Morvill who encountered difficulties in providing sound foundations for the piers, owing to the depth of the loose gravel which had to be removed. However, he made a first class job of it, but lost money. He did, in recognition of his good workmanship, receive a special grant of £40 from the West Riding Justices at Pontefract. In due time, this lovely bridge will be relieved of the heavy traffic when the Aire Valley trunk road becomes a complete reality.

Before we reach Apperley, it is worthwhile making our way to the tow-path of the Leeds/Liverpool canal, and following it to the spot where the canal crosses the Aire by means of a bridge of no less than seven stone arches, which seem just as safe and secure today as when they were built, some two hundred years ago. Another feat of 18th century civil engineering.

APPERLEY BRIDGE

Here we have a bridge connecting two inns, the George and Dragon and the Stansfield Arms. The latter is named after the family of that name who lived at Esholt Hall, subsequent to Sir Walter Calverley who built the residence. The inn was originally the gatehouse of the Hall. Opposite the inn is the well-known Woodhouse Grove School, founded in 1812 for the education of Wesleyan ministers' sons, the first tutor being a Mr Fennell. A curious anomaly here, for a local Quaker, Robert Elam, who once owned the property, thought fit to erect the round tower which still stands on a wooded knoll near the school. This tower frequently attracts attention from close quarters and is known as Elam's Temple, and Elam felt it was an appropriate place for distributing charity. To attract and absorb as much labour as possible, he arranged for the building stones to be carried from their source to the site.

As regards the bridge, one Nigel Plumpton gave, in 1189, the fishing rights in the river Aire to the Nunnery at Esholt, providing they kept the wooden bridge at Apperley in repair. The rights extended from Apperley to a point in Shipley where the Bradford Beck joined the Aire – a fine stretch indeed in 1190. At that time, no bridge existed between Bingley and Kirkstall (some 14 miles). The next we hear about the bridge is that, on 1st August 1366, Henry Casteley of Ottelay and Agnes, his wife, conveyed to Richard del Grene of Eshold, three acres of land and waste in the clearing called le Birggrode which was bounded on one side by "The King's highway leading to the brigg at Apperley". Some 300 years later, lands, meadows, woods and pasture in the clearing (Briggerode) lying on the eastern side of Apperleybrigg, which had been held by Thomas del Idle, later vicar of 'Calverle' by gift of John Adamson of Otley, were conveyed to Nicholas Adamson of Otley, chaplain, apparently son of John Adamson, the original donor.

The nunnery is no more, of course, and the Hall at Esholt with its low-lying meadows eventually became the site of the Bradford Corporation's model sewage disposal plant, which was well ahead of so many other undertakings of this kind.

With the dissolution of the monasteries, it would seem that the bridge would be seriously wanting in repair, but we do know that the crossing was in existence as a stone affair towards the end of the 16th century. However, it is on record that it was in such a poor state of repair that a Thomas Walmsley of Bolton by Bowland (a builder of high repute) was commissioned to rebuilt it. A price of £99 was agreed and paid in instalments over a period of twelve months, and on 26th June 1602 he received the final instalment of £39 when the bridge was completed. It must be said that the stone and other materials required were provided for him, but he agreed to come from Bolton by Bowland from time to time, to do any repairs that were necessary for the sum of 5/- per annum as long as he lived. To agree to this speaks well of the man's confidence in the high workmanship he put into the structure.

We are not certain of the age of Thomas Walmsley at the date of his death, but by 1669 repairs began to be necessary over a period of 35 years. Sir Walter Calverley attended Wakefield Sessions c 1700 and secured more money for repairs. Samuel Hemmingway of the nearby George and Dragon Inn also received money for repairs, and bridge stones and rails for use when the water level was over the bridge ends.

The George and Dragon, probably the oldest in the district, possesses no little amount of interest. The stone set into the gable of the east end of the inn bears the date '1704', the year of its enlargement by Samuel Hemming-way, and it would appear from that, and the inscription cut in the large stone built into the outer wall of the large ground floor bar, that previous in 1704, it had been a place of refreshment. The inscription is in Latin, but the following translation appears below the stone and reads:

> 'Not for the purpose of making a show, but for necessary uses, Samuel Hemmingway and his wife Mary enlarged this house AD 1704 (MDCCIV). These things are cherishing: victuals, drink, warmth, shelter which, if thou possess, remember gratefully to give thanks to God.'
> The property belonged to the Hemmingway family of Bradford for very many years.

Some say that, at one time, when there was no bridge, and the river was crossed by means of a ford, the inn was the old ford house. In view of records of a bridge as far back as 1190, we can only assume that the bridge must have been unsafe for a period of years and so a crossing was made by means of a ford.

Before leaving the inn, one must not miss the special curiosity to be seen inside. Many years ago, a large oak tree grew – not outside, but inside. The huge trunk is there for all to see in the main bar. Be assured that the branches are not pushing their way through the roof. It is not now living, of course, but it genuinely rises out of the floor. The original bark has long since gone – wear, tear and decay – but has been replaced with genuine bark of an old oak tree felled some years ago in Sherwood Forest.

Across the bridge they all came. Scotch drapers, well-to-do and not so well-to-do businessmen, and travellers of all classes sought refreshment at this pleasant port of call. Even half of Fairfax's army crossed the bridge in 1643 in the Civil War days, as the Royalists had destroyed Kirkstall Bridge.

The bridge as it stands today is a lovely old stone affair of two large segmental arches and a central cutwater. Two modest-sized vehicles can just squeeze past each other if they meet. There is no sidewalk and the roads from Idle and Rawdon both make a decided swing to approach it. In spite of the ceaseless traffic on the massive modern bridge a short way downstream, motor cars cross and recross the old one, some of them stopping at the ancient hostelry for refreshment, as they did centuries ago on foot or by horse.

A priceless gem of an inscription carved on a stone tablet can be seen on the east parapet. It used to read:

> (Sir Walter) Calverley, bart, claimeth halfe this (Bridge) and the waste ground at the south side of the Bridge to the said side of the Brook it being his right as Lord of the Manor of Idle.

Unfortunately the top third of the tablet has been allowed to flake away.

We cannot leave Apperley Bridge without recalling an unusual incident which happened on 29th February 1824. The so-called prophet, John Roe, vowed he had had a vision, and so founded a sect called Jerusalemites. His powers, said to have been given by our Lord, would enable him to walk dryshod across the river Aire. On the river banks and on the bridge an enormous crowd assembled and awaited the ceremonious arrival of John Roe.

The waters of the Aire neither supported John's weight, nor did they part. Fortunately, he and his followers suffered no more than a mud and water bath. He was born in Bowling, Bradford, and baptised in the Parish Church (now the Cathedral). He was a bankrupt before he took up trading on the credulous. He died in Australia after setting up 'temples' in Oldham and in Wakefield.

CASTLEFORD AND ITS RIVER CROSSING

Today, a visitor to Castleford, either on business or to see a rugby league match, coming shopping or just passing through, could be excused for being quite unaware of its ancient and quite remarkable past. Even the old parish church was recast in the 19th century. Surrounding the town are chemical and glass works as well as heavy industries.

"Where's the Roman Fort?" a few may ask on arrival at Castleford.

"There's nothing to see."

"Yes, but where's the site?"

"Well, you go through Leo's Supermarket and down to the foot of their car park, and on your left, you'll see a neatly kept area of grass – that's the site of the Roman Regimental Bath House."

And for confirmation, there is a large clean block of stone at the north-west corner. On it there is a circular plaque with gold lettering on a maroon ground, bearing the legend:

CASTLEFORD AND DISTRICT CIVIC TRUST
The Roman Bath-house in this area.
Archaeological excavations in 1978
revealed the well-preserved remains
of the Military Bath-house of a
Roman auxilliary fort.

One stands there and wonders where the main fort once stood. For its exact position, one needs to retrace one's steps, turn left into Carlton Street and on the right hand of the pedestrianised section is a specially-erected post, with a framed plan showing its exact position and brief notes of Castleford's Roman history. Underneath that large car park, then, Roman soldiers once ate, slept, exercised and played table games.

The river was forded, surely, just north of the fort, but a wee bit upstream. Castleford – castra (fort) near the ford – was known as Legentium in Roman times. The Roman road ran just west of the fort and down to the river, crossed the latter and made its way to the north and Aberford and beyond, but our object is to have more than a look at the 'modern' bridge over the river Aire; however, on the way along Aire Street, we must surely pause at a large building bearing a prominent sign proclaiming it as the world's largest stone-grinding flour mill. Small parties can be shown round, on application, and see for themselves the fascinating work that goes on there.

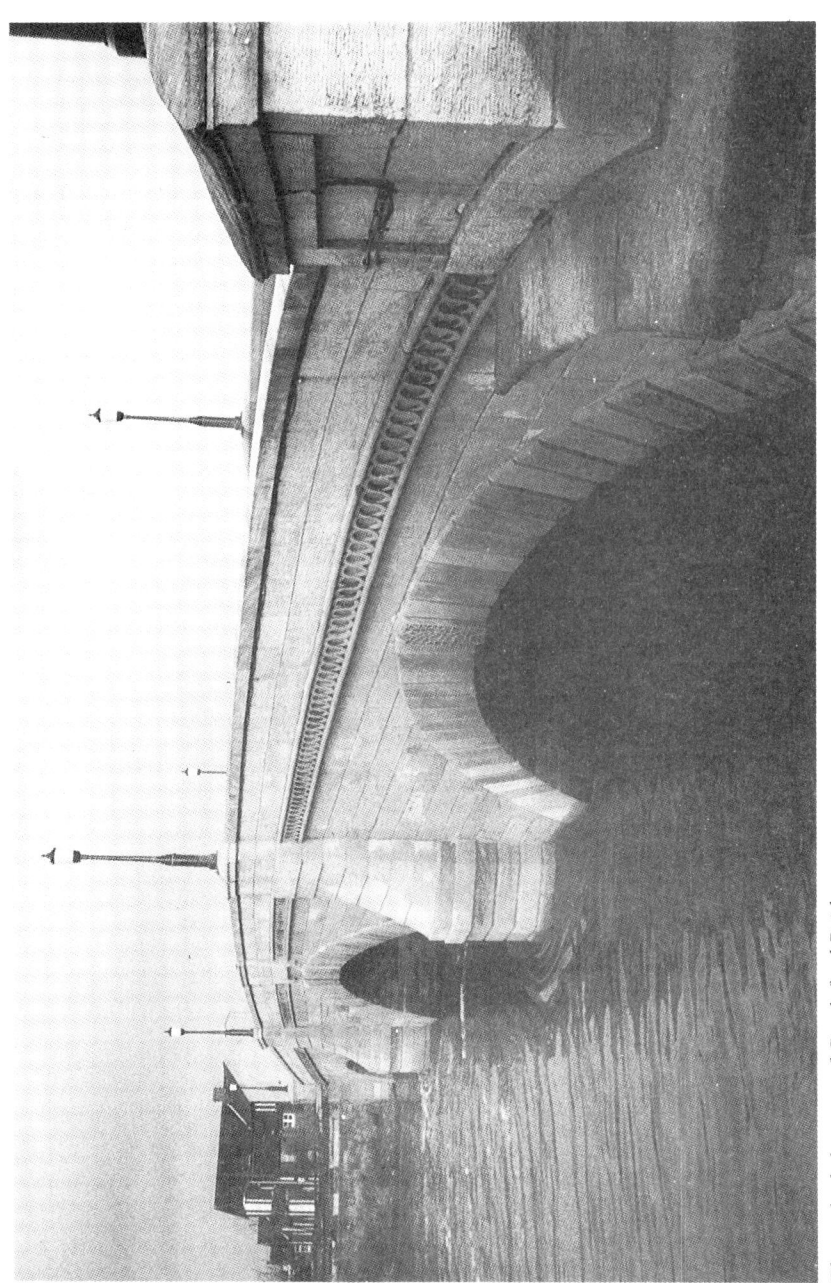

The arched elegance of Castleford Bridge

Just a couple of hundred yards or so along Aire Street brings one to the bridge, which takes modern traffic to join Ermine Street and later the Great North Road.

This bridge, of three beautifully proportioned arches of mellow sandstone, carries a none too wide roadway over the Aire, which is now a river of some size, having been joined by the Calder a little upstream. Vehicles passing over the bridge are controlled by traffic lights.

The bridge is almost 190 years old, and reflects the skill and, indeed, the rather special ability of the architect and builder. The west and east parapets respectively perpetuate this with carved stone plaques:

BERNARD HARTLEY
ARCHITECT
1805

JESSE HARTLEY
BUILDER
1808

Each outer parapet of the bridge has a string of carved rings in the stonework from one end to the other, adding a touch of artistry whilst retaining the elegance of the whole.

Looking over the parapet to the foot of the bridge, one sees some stone steps rising from the water's edge, and pictures the days when passengers could be seen disembarking from the river-then-sea-then-river service from London, via Goole. Passengers changed to stage coach to, say, Leeds and the West Riding, to quicken the already tedious journey by water. Those stone steps were used to enable passengers to reach the top of the steep river bank to board the waiting coach, and so Castleford became an important stopping place. In the 18th and 19th centuries canals, of course, among other things, became important connecting links between river and river, especially in this historic part of Yorkshire.

To obtain a good frontal view of the bridge from the west, one must descend an alleyway near a fruit and vegetable market. The alley contains much flotsam and jetsam, not all of which has been brought down by the river in flood! It is well worthwhile, however, to make one's way down to the water's edge to obtain the view.

Apart from the Romans, who crossed the river upstream, there have been many historic occasions at Castleford. The Danes sallied from York and defeated King Edred's army there in AD 948, as the King was returning south after having ravaged Northumbria. As soon as things settled down after this, Northumbria ceased to be a separate kingdom from England.

William the Conqueror's advance north towards York was halted at Castleford for three weeks, owing to the flooded state of the Aire. A crossing was not possible, either by boat or ferry. Whilst waiting for the flood waters to abate, the redoubtable William got around a bit, and noted the importance of the site which is now Pontefract.

The first bridge appears to have been erected towards the middle of the 12th century – a wooden one. The present one replaced an ancient seven-arched stone affair which the famous Royal Antiquary, Leland, passed over in c 1530. Some 275 years later, like many bridges in the 16th and 17th centuries which had come to be in a 'ruinous' state and, in spite of many repairs over the years, needed really serious attention, the old Castleford Bridge was demolished and completely rebuilt.

FERRYBRIDGE

The last of our bridges over the Aire only two and a half miles downstream from Castleford, eventually became a far more important crossing, as it carried an ever increasing amount of traffic on what was to become the Great North Road.

In the Domesday Book the village of Ferrybridge was referred to as Ferie, and about one hundred years later as Feria. Although there does not appear any record of a ferry in existence at that time, there may well have been one. About AD 1290, however, it seems that a bridge was built, and a priest was appointed in AD 1306 to the Chapel of St Mary at 'Fery juxta pontem', and tolls collected. Possibly the then landowners (de Lacies) used the money, or at least some of it, to maintain the bridge. Soon after that (AD 1314) we learn that 'indulgences were granted to those making or repairing the causeway between Brotherton and Feribrig'.

A large tract of very flat land has existed from time immemorial on the northern bank of the Aire from Knottingley to Brotherton, and is still known as the Brotherton Marshes; it seems obvious that some sort of raised causeway was necessary to cross the marshes from Ferrybridge to Brotherton, especially in the winter.

We hear that Queen Margaret (second wife of Edward I), when staying at Pontefract Castle in AD 1300, was crossing the marshes, perhaps on the causeway, when she went into labour. She was rushed to the Manor House at Brotherton, which had been the one-time residence of the Archbishop of York. The Queen gave birth to a son, who was named Thomas de Brotherton. In AD 1312, Thomas was created Earl of Norfolk by Edward II, and subsequently became Marshall of England, the ancestor of subsequent Dukes of Norfolk. The present Manor House dates from AD 1664 and was built on the site of the original, and when we visit or read about that enormous stronghold, Arundel Castle in Sussex, it is nice to remember that the first Duke of Norfolk was born in that little village in Yorkshire.

Before we traverse the marshes on foot to Brotherton, let us have a good look at the bridge at Ferrybridge. Approaching it from the village's main street, we turn left and behold an enormous concrete arch spanning the river, but framed by this arch is a three-arched stone bridge of beautiful proportions. The south approach is supported by four small arches, one of which is blocked with silt and stones. Most of the north approach is buried under the embankment supporting the Great North Road. One small arch is visible, however. Balustrades adorn the east and west parapets but plain stonework faces the old carriageway. Here again, one sees the work of

Bernard Hartley of Pontefract recorded on a large stone plaque, dated 1804, and on the opposite parapet is the name John Carr, Esq of York, Architect 1797. John Carr was, of course, associated with many bridges and buildings in Yorkshire, as previously mentioned.

The bridge which carried the Great North Road for so many years is now blocked at the northern end, and only foot passengers can gain access to the other side of the river. Large stone flags now cover the greater part of the former carriageway. A fascinating domicile near the approach to the bridge from the south is Toll Bridge House. It stands in splendid isolation, and the lady of the house tells me that, as a toll house, it dates back to the reign of Charles I (1600–1649) and is a listed property, grade three. Inside it is quite unique, but beware of the dogs!

Nearby is the only surviving inn by the bridge – the Golden Lion – and a little downstream, where the river makes a graceful bend, the first lock appears and gives access to the Aire and Calder navigation canal. Gone are the two other famous inns, the Angel and the Swan, on the south and north sides of the river respectively. In connection with the Angel, there was an exciting but sad episode which is worth recording:

> 'A gentleman travelling in a postchaise had accidentally left an empty purse on a table in one of the rooms. When the mistake was discovered a man was sent off to overtake and return him his property. When he came near to the chaise, he imprudently called out stop, your purse, your purse! on which the gentleman believing that a highwayman was demanding his purse shot him dead and drove on. Afterwards, on being informed of his fatal mistake, it is said he liberally provided for the widow and children. This was in 1781'.

The inns provided first class accommodation and Ferrybridge became one of the main posting houses on the Great North Road. Some 20 to 30 stage coaches passed this way every day, and vehicles of all descriptions stopped here as well as the travellers, many of the nobility, coachmen, guards, postillions, postboys, grooms and porters. All needed to be catered for.

Gone, alas, the old pottery and the glass bottle factory which once occupied the north bank of the Aire near the bridge. The new monster bridge occupies a large slice of land where these old firms once plied their trade, and carries thousands of vehicles of all shapes and sizes, which thunder their way north and south in never-ending stream all day and far into the night.

So, let us now make our way to Brotherton from Ferrybridge bridge.

There is a choice of paths. One leads from the bridge and up the embankment of the new Great North Road to a paved footway adjacent to the road. The other drops down to the river bank to a slightly raised pathway leading to the slip road to lower Brotherton.

Either walk is interesting. The riverside path gives one a close-up view of large barges making their way up and down the river, and through those graceful arches of the Carr and Hartley Bridge. Incidentally, local people assert that the foundations of the bridge are laid on bales of cotton. Fascinating!

Taking the riverside path, then, we can see what our old friend, Leland, meant when he recorded his visit in 1538, regarding the marshes:

"A Causey of stone with divers bridges over it [the marsh]
to drean the Low Meadow Water on the left Hand in Aire
River about a mile to Ferry-Bridge."

These bridges are still shown on the modern 6" Ordnance Survey maps. High above them, on the embankment, thunders the ceaseless traffic, of today.

The path adjacent to the Great North Road gives one a view, not only of the 'Little Marsh', but of the much larger low-lying land to the east, where one can picture the Battle of Brotherton taking place, when the Yorkists routed the Lancastrians. A common fighting ground it was, too, during the Wars of the Roses and the rivalry for possession of the crossing at Ferrybridge.

In 1530, Cardinal Wolsey, out of favour with Henry VIII, was ordered to Cawood Castle. It was at this time that he is said to have confirmed hundreds of children on his way from Cawood. Many were assembled at a great cross of stone near Ferrybridge. This suggests a spot on Brotherton Marsh near the North Road, but no stone or remains of a cross can now be seen.

Wolsey was sent to London after he was arrested for high treason, but never reached there as he died at Leicester, on the way to his trial.

On this sad note, we end our travels in the Aire valley, and have a look at Calderdale.

CALDERDALE

Of all the Yorkshire Dales, Calderdale is one which most of us rarely think of as being a tourist area, yet it possesses some rare gems. All too often one associates it with those 'dark satanic mills', a few of which are derelict due to declining trade. Others have been brought to life with new industries, and some have been demolished, but it is often forgotten that at least a few industrial towns have a history dating back to the Norman Conquest, if not Roman times.

Where are the gems, then?

I pick out three quite unique bridges as a start. The first is at Hebden Bridge; this rather special Pennine town is situated at the confluence of Hebden Water and the River Calder, and the steep-sided hills forming the two valleys come right down to the water, except for a few acres near the confluence. There are many points of interest at Hebden Bridge, as the visitor will soon realize if he takes the trouble to call at the Information Centre, but in this book we are mainly concerned with the ancient packhorse bridge and its adjacent arch. Hebden Water, which has its source some way beyond Hardcastle Crags, a well-wooded and lengthy valley and local beauty spot, enters the town from the north, and flows through its middle to join the Calder, just before the latter passes under the arches holding up the Rochdale Canal at the southern end of the town. Here is another example of 18th century civil engineering skills.

The four old packhorse routes from Halifax, Rochdale, Heptonstall and Burnley met at Hebden Bridge, and crossed Hebden Water by means of the bridge which still stands, little changed since 1510. It consists of three arches, under two of which flows Hebden water. The third arch allowed the passage of 'used' water, after it had worked the wheel at the one-time manorial corn mill of Wadsworth, the site of which was near the present St George's Bridge (1892/3, built of cast iron with stone embellishment in the centre of the parapet) and just a little upstream from the packhorse bridge.

The modern approach from Bridgegate to the old bridge has been very well planned; it is well-flagged on two levels, and there is seating. Young children, often accompanied by an adult, come with pieces of bread and feed the mallards and pigeons – a pleasant sight with the old bridge in the background, especially in the sunshine. The bridge is, of course, closed to motor cars and the like. In any case, it is too narrow for such vehicles, but on crossing it on foot one is led to the famous hostelry, 'The Hole in the Wall', rebuilt alas! It has, like the bridge, an eventful history, being at the junction of the packhorse routes. Its name is said to have originated from the battering it had in the Civil War days. On this, the west side, there is a pleasant open space with a weeping willow backed with a well-built wall, with stone features and a seat at the foot, which affords an attractive view of the bridge. From here one can ascend the steep hillside to Heptonstall, an absolute museum piece of a village of one-time hand looms. In addition to the village pump and the remains of stocks, there are the oldest cloth hall in Yorkshire and oldest Wesleyan chapel in the world, the foundation stone of which was laid by John Wesley nearly 240 years ago. The remains of the old church are full of interest, too.

But to return to the packhorse bridge. There is a well-made plaque on the side of Hebden Water, near the bridge itself, which gives a brief history:

HEBDEN OLD BRIDGE ERECTED CIRCA AD 1510
REPLACING A MEDIEVAL BRIDGE BUILT OF
TIMBER

MANY REPAIRS WERE NECESSARY IN AD 1602
AND AGAIN IN AD 1657, THE PARAPET BEING
REPAIRED IN AD 1845 AND RAISED IN AD 1890

THE EASTERN ARCH OF THE BRIDGE SPANS THE
TAIL GOIT OF BRIDGE MILL, ORIGINALLY THE
MANORIAL CORN MILL OF WADSWORTH

Quaint snippets of history can be gleaned from the several inscriptions carved in stone on the bridge itself, and the oldest are those of AD 1602 and AD 1657 on the north parapet facing upstream. They can be seen at close quarters from the flat wall top approaching the bridge, but care needs to be taken to avoid the prickly shrubbery which tends to discourage one.

It is interesting to note that in 1508, a James Grenewode of nearby Wadsworth left the princely sum of 3 s: 4d for the fabric of a stone bridge, and a Wm Murgatroyd left in the same year the sum of 6 s: 8d for the same purpose (10 s: 8d in all). By 1510 a further 13 s: 4d had been left by Wm Grenewode and 6 s: 8d by Richard Naylor, making a grand total of £2.

A devotee of the Brontë family, who wishes to make a diversion to have a look at Hebden Bridge, should follow the interesting route via Oxenhope over wild Pennine heights to the fantastic descent into the town – he will remember it well.

To discover the second gem, one must follow the Halifax road as far as the right-hand turning for Sowerby Bridge, make another very steep descent to the traffic lights, and turn right again for Ripponden, three miles, along a well-wooded valley up the river Ryburn, an important tributary of the Calder. At Ripponden is a quadruple gem of antiquity. A unique inn, a packhorse bridge, a church and a quaint corner of domestic property are clustered together.

RIPPONDEN

Surprising, quaint, picturesque, ancient . . . one could go on and on. Where in Yorkshire, or anywhere else, can one find a gilded packhorse bridge, which leads one straight over the river to a really ancient inn which bears no name or inn sign? Only in the Ryburn Valley, which carries a major tributary of the Calder. The church of St Bartholomew stands in the same relative position as that at Hubberholme in Wharfedale with its church and inn. Gilded? Well, the stone parapets are fairly low, and protection of the traveller is afforded by means of black-painted dwarf iron railings with gilded terminals. Somehow, they do not seem to detract from the bridge's appeal. The only thing which does detract is the ugly drain pipe which crosses the river, above water level, in normal conditions. It is right under the bridge. The landlord of the inn says that the original pipe was swept away in a great flood, and the local council replaced it with one, not just as ugly, but much bigger!

I am indebted to Timothy Walker at the inn for a great deal of information about the inn, the bridge and the church.

The Old Bridge Inn, as it is known, is one of Yorkshire's oldest hostelries, and it is not hard to imagine yourself in another age when you look down to it, with its bridge and church, from a vantage point on the 'new road' (B 6113) leading to Greetland, Elland and the south. The old road passed the door of the inn, over the packhorse bridge (an ancient monument) and then the church to climb the steep hill (Ripponden Bank). As in the case of the Blue Bell Inn at nearby Soyland, it is generally accepted that the Romans passed this way on their journeys between York and Chester via Blackstone Edge, crossing the River Ryburn at Ripponden by the ford at what is known as Brigroyd.

First mentioned in a document dated October 18th, 1313, the inn is believed to have been a church-owned monastic guest house – a theory supported by the pilgrim's crosses engraved on stone inside the building. During excavations by the owners in 1963, an ancient font, thought to be pre-reformation, was unearthed from the car park. Presumably it came from the early church, and is there to be seen by all in the inn itself. Early panelling, a daub and wattle wall and a fine cruck beam were discovered during restoration work. At the present time, there are two levels. In the centre of the building is the bar area, and passing the old font, you go down a few steps to the oak-beamed dining room and buffet bar. To the left of the main bar area is an oak panelled public room, and under this a fine vaulted cellar. It is interesting to find that, from the room above the latter, a few

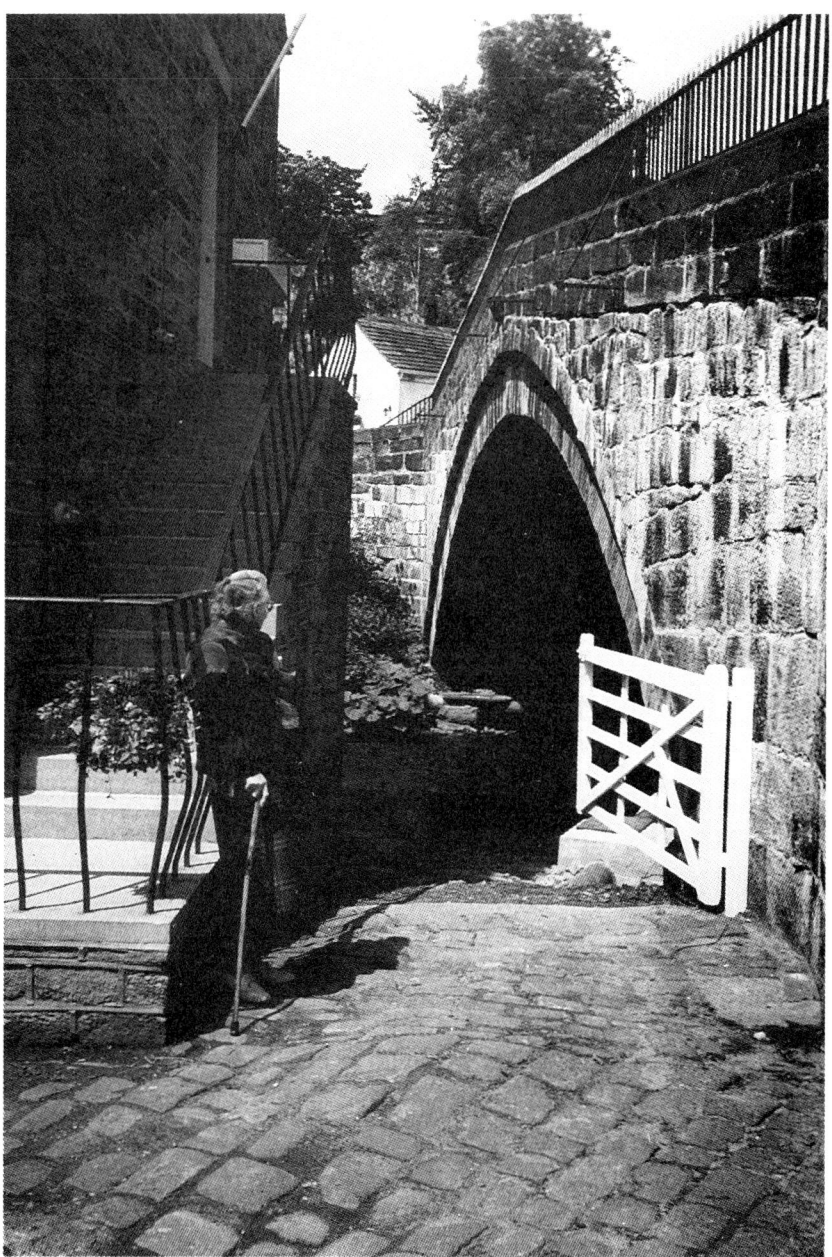

The packhorse bridge at Ripponden

steps up lead to a door in the panelling. This door gives way to a store room, in which I was shown the wall displaying daub and wattle, about which it was stated that a piece of lime taken from it consisted of no less than 250 layers! Little is known of the precise history of the inn before 1700, as most of the parish records were lost in 1722, when the old Ripponden church was destroyed by flood. The church was rebuilt in 1737, but subsequent repairs proved so costly that it was pulled down and another built on the same site in 1866/68. This is the church of St Bartholomew which stands there today.

The owner of the inn about that time was the famous Samuel Hill of Making Place in Soyland. Hill had become wealthy as a far-sighted manufacturer of worsted cloths, which he exported to the continent throughout the first half of the 18th century. Records show that Hill had as many as 90 packhorses at a time, travelling on this route to the ports, and he himself is known to have been a regular caller at the inn, which seems to have been occupied by tenant landlords.

An actual reference to an innkeeper occurs in 1754, when the inn was described as the (ale) house of Richard Hirstwood. He was succeeded in 1798 by John Schofield, whose widow, Hannah, took over in 1814, to be succeeded in turn by her daughter, Ruth. During Hannah's time, the inn was renamed the Waterloo to commemorate Wellington's victory over Napoleon, and in some quarters locally it is still referred to by that name. Ruth was known colloquially in her day as Ruth o' t' Waterloo.

Like the inn, the first record of a bridge was in 1313. It would, of course, have been built of wood as likely as not, but in 1533, William Firth of Field House, Sowerby left the sum of 7s:6d for the building of a stone bridge!

Ripponden folk are strong-minded, and when a one-time landlord of the inn fell out with the church folk, he declared that, rather than let them use the bridge, he would pull it down; it was his anyway, he said, since he had paid a fine of £10. Without arguing the strange logic of the matter, the then rector raised £10, gave it to the landlord and declared the matter settled.

Ripponden somehow entwines itself into the history of England. Daniel Defoe is said to have stayed at the Old Bridge Inn in the 1720s en route to Halifax, quite coincidentally, where he embarked on the writing of Robinson Crusoe. Some years later, a writer of a different stamp was busy in Ripponden. He was the incumbent of the time, a Mr Watson, whose History of Halifax would be a priceless find today for a fortunate collector.

John Collier, the famous Lancashire poet and artist (known as Tim Bobbin), had some lively times at the Old Bridge Inn, in between lettering stones in the nearby churchyard in the 18th century. He painted many inn signs throughout Yorkshire and Cheshire. His legacy, in the form of a self-portrait, used to hang in the bar, but was moved 'next door' some years ago, as pipe tobacco and cigarette smoke 'didn't do it any good'. A good reason. If Tim Bobbin painted a sign for the inn, there doesn't seem to be any evidence of it being hung. Strange.

It is hard to tear oneself away from this corner of Ripponden, but we must get along to the jewel in the crown – the Chantry Bridge over the Calder at Wakefield.

CITY OF WAKEFIELD AND ITS CHANTRY BRIDGE

Wakefield – once the chief medieval town in the old West Riding of Yorkshire. It was one of the manors held by the Archbishop of York along with Otley and Ripon, and can claim a very eventful history dating back to before the Conquest. Edward the Confessor, crowned in 1041, was by far the largest landowner in Yorkshire.

Entering an industrial West Yorkshire town or city can be a depressing experience, but entering Wakefield from Bradford, one is at once impressed with the 18th century mellow red-brick terraces and detached houses. Thousands of the older generations of motorists will remember the famous address: No 14, St John's North, but how many actually went there and saw that long and beautiful terrace of houses with white porticos. Incidentally, the name plate on No 14 now reads 'West Yorkshire Archaeological Service'. On the other side of the main road is St John's Church, built in 1781 of smooth Yorkshire stone, and placed in the middle of one side of a huge square of greensward, with dignified red-brick terraces and houses, again with white porticos.

A little nearer the centre of the city is the magnificent County Hall, circa 1898. Its interior is, perhaps, just as magnificent as the exterior. The stone arches in the large entrance hall impress one very much. Then we come to the Crown Court, with its six Doric columns and pediment in Adam style with garlands, Royal Arms and dome-roofed tower. The interior, which can be inspected, is a splendid example of the dignity of the 1830s.

As we make our way down to the river very slowly, we cannot fail to stop and look inside the Town Hall, which, in addition to the normal offices, houses, without ostentation, an Information Centre and a third-floor Clock Tower restaurant and lounge, both very dignified, and formerly the Council members' dining area. Next down the street is the old Mechanics Institution, now the City Museum.

Just a little out of our way to the Bridge and Chantry Chapel is a one-storey Elizabethan building, with the following inscription on the stonework:

> SCHOLA REGINAE ELIZABETH I
> BUILDED BY GEORGE SAVILE AND
> GEORGE SAVILE THOMAS SAVILE
> ESQUIRE HIS SONNES

It was, of course, the old Elizabethan Grammar School of 1590. It is now The Elizabethan Gallery and opens its doors for exhibitions.

We must now make our way to the river, and on the return journey inspect the Cathedral and Ridings shopping centre, as well as South Parade and Westgate. From many parts of the old West Riding, motor traffic used to come this way to cross the river by means of the ancient bridge over the Calder, and then on to Doncaster and the Great North Road. Now, of course the enormously increased amount of traffic crossing the river means that the old bridge has had to be bypassed. A massive concrete and steel affair takes its place, and is approached by a new road to the north of the cathedral.

If the modern motorist desires to pause awhile on his journey on an almost deserted stretch of road, he will leave the southbound carriageway soon after passing under the railway bridge, and turning left he will see the nine-arched bridge of sand-coloured stone. On it stands the Chantry Chapel of St Mary on the Bridge. There is no parking on the bridge itself, but at the time of writing there is ample space just before reaching it.

On the eastern parapet, the Rotary Club of Wakefield Chantry has erected a plaque, which reads:

THIS STONE BRIDGE, BUILT SOON AFTER 1342,
REPLACED AN EARLIER BRIDGE OVER THE RIVER
CALDER. THE PACKHORSE BRIDGE WAS ADDED IN
1730 AND 1797. THE CHANTRY CHAPEL OF ST.
MARY, BUILT BETWEEN 1342 AND 1356, IS ONE OF
ONLY FOUR CHAPELS SURVIVING IN ENGLAND. IT
WAS RESTORED IN 1847 AND MORE RECENTLY.

The other chantry chapels still intact in England are, of course at Rother-ham (Yorkshire), St Ives, Huntingdonshire (Cambs) and Bradford on Avon, Somerset (Avon).

This gem of antiquity, integral with its bridge, stands there serenely, in spite of its wholly industrial surroundings, quite unique, with the possible exception of Rotherham.

It should be mentioned that Wakefield's chapel is under the care of the parish of St Andrew, which provides services. Many efforts have been made to attract tourists, with only initial success. However, a charitable body – 'The Friends of the Chantry Chapel, Wakefield' – has been formed and officially launched; in a colourful ceremony on 8th September 1991, the chairman of the Friends, Mr J Gilbey, introduced the Lord Mayor and Lady St Oswald of Nostell Priory, who made appropriate speeches in front of the west front of the chapel. The object is to raise funds for maintenance, and to publicise its attractiveness, as well as encourage membership of the Friends (Secretary – Mr RF Perraudin, 2 Westfield Park, Wakefield).

Services are held as follows: Holy Communion, first Sunday in the month, and Evening Prayer on the third Sunday, both at 3 pm.

The interior is perfect. The old font is kept near the entrance as a reminder that it is the beginning of life within the Christian Church. The east window seems wider than it appears from the outside; its main features are the Annunciation, Elizabeth greeting Mary, the Birth of Jesus, the Wise Men, the Crucifixion, the Lamb of God, the Burial of Christ, the Resurrection, the Ascension and the Coming of the Holy Ghost.

The carved stone heads on the side of the window represent Edward III and Queen Philippa, in whose reign the bridge is said to have been built. In the north-east corner, a small door leads to a spiral staircase up to the bell tower, near the top of which is a tiny window which gives a view of the interior of the chapel, especially the entrance, so that there was liaison between the bell-ringer and the warden, as to when the latter was to close the doors. At the top of the staircase is another door, which leads to the roof. The spiral staircase also descends to the crypt, used as a robing room. One important feature of the crypt is the outline of a former doorway, giving direct access to the island on which the chapel stands, although most of the west wall of the crypt is integral with the bridge. Fishing took place from here, and tolls from the river traffic were taken.

Back in the chapel itself, the visitor should note the cross-beam of oak, with its inscription in Latin which tells us that 'The word was made flesh. Glory to God in the Highest'.

The west front, facing the roadway, has had an eventful history. The present façade dates from 1940. The first one was replaced in 1847, but the stone then used was quite soft, and weathered so badly that it was removed and re-erected near the lake in the grounds of Kettlethorpe Hall. Kettlethorpe Hall Park is to be found by the side of the Barnsley road, just before reaching Pledwick Well Inn. It is open to the public.

The bridge itself should be viewed from both the east and west sides. On the west side, the arches are rounded and support the widened carriageway (still fairly narrow), but viewed from the east side, pointed arches will be noted, and display antiquity. To obtain a lovely view of the bridge and chapel, it is recommended that the visitor should cross it from the north side to the south, and bear left, under the arches of a miniature bridge of stone, to the greensward with seats. Follow the river bank for about a hundred yards, then look upstream.

Back on the bridge admiring the intricate carving of the west front of the chapel, one cannot fail to picture the famous Battle of Wakefield in December 1460, which occurred in the fields between the Chantry and nearby Sandal Castle scant remains of which can still be seen. The castle was the headquarters of the Duke of York. The latter's blood being raised to battling point, he sallied forth and fell into the hands of the Lancastrians who showed no mercy, the Duke's bravery being of no avail.

Then came Henry VIII and the Dissolution, and in 1548 the Chantry was sold for 55/- in 11 annual instalments of 5/- (0% interest!). In 1553/1558 (Queen Mary) the Chantry was re-opened for worship, but by 1727 it was being used as a warehouse, and later as a newsroom. Final restoration took place in April 1971, and it was re-opened by Bishop Treacy, assisted by Bishop Ramsbottom and the Rev G T Willett.

The cathedral church of All Saints, which now stands free from the noise of ceaseless motor traffic, as pedestrian precincts surround it, is 500 years old for the most part. The 247 ft spire is the highest in Yorkshire. Many parts of the cathedral are much older, and it is well worthwhile purchasing a modestly-priced guide from the bookshop therein. Just outside is the Bishop Treacy Memorial Hall – a fitting reminder of the great character who was Bishop from 1968 to his death in 1978. Whilst on the subject of clergy, the name of Oliver Goldsmith comes to mind. His novel, The Vicar of Wakefield, is one of his best known, if not actually read – a delightful story indeed. Goldsmith must have been greatly impressed with Wakefield as it was in the 18th century.

Before we leave Wakefield altogether, No 136 Westgate is worth examining. It has a beautiful 18th century porch, with a frieze in Adam style with garlands. It is just down the street from the railway station, and just above the station is a unique 18th century Unitarian chapel, with a frontage of symmetry and grace.

South Parade is a terrace dated 1775 and faces a green. Each house has an attractive doorway and iron balconies. Another reminder of Wakefield's graceful past.

ROTHERHAM

A town whose history goes back far beyond that of many others in England.

Apart from Bronze Age and Iron Age relics found in the vicinity, there is much evidence of Roman occupation from AD 54. A visit to Clifton Park and Museum near the centre of the town – a few minutes' walk from the great church of All Saints – will reward the visitor with a view of the remains of the colonnade of the Granary and columns of the portico of the Roman Fort. Actually, they are re-erections of the original stonework 'rescued' when industry threatened to destroy them elsewhere in Rotherham. Other relics are to be seen in the Museum itself.

Following the Conquest of 1066, the Domesday Book records that a church was being built in RODERHAM (1074), but the Vicar of Rotherham tells me that a church stood on the site as early as 937, and that a Norman church was built on the old foundations in the 12th century. The lands passed to the Cistercians of Rufford, who pulled down the Norman church and erected one in the perpendicular style in the 15th century, but the nave arch and chancel arch display Norman stonework. The present magnificent church dominates the town centre, and from the river the pedestrian approach to it, with its fountains and beds of flowers, belies the fact that the town is very industrialized 'just round the corner'.

The Archbishop of York in 1480 was none other than Thomas Rotherham; he was born in what is now called College Street in the centre of the town. It was he who founded the College of Jesus in Rotherham in the late 15th century, and, in the following year, the Chantry Chapel on the bridge over the river Don. The expense was largely borne by him. He was also Chancellor of England. From the time the Chapel was built until Henry VIII closed it, it was used by travellers over the bridge to ask for God's blessing upon their journeys, and masses were said for the repose of the dead.

From its closure onwards, the Chapel of our Lady had a chequered career. At first it was converted into an almshouse, but in 1779 it became a deputy constable's house, and prisoners were kept in the crypt. For some time after that it was used solely as the constable's residence. In 1888, it was turned into a newsagent's and tobacconist's shop. Fortunately, the people of Rotherham were unhappy at this desecration of such a sacred place, but it took many years and much hard work before the Chapel was restored and re-dedicated in 1924. Since then, further restoration has taken place. Of special note is the east window, incorporated in the stained glass of which is the coat of arms of Thomas Rotherham. The window also reflects quite vividly God's presence throughout the Chapel's history as well as the little statue of Our Lady. The latter is modern, and replaces one which was removed at the Dissolution in 1547. It is a gentle reminder of the chapel's dedication. I am indebted to the Vicar of Rotherham, Rev S G N Brindley, who not only gave me so much information, but specially opened up the chantry chapel for my visit. On entering, one is immediately impressed by the beauty of the place, duly complemented by the obvious care and attention given to keeping it immaculate. High quality is evident whichever way one looks. A descent into the crypt is made through a trap door in the floor of the chapel near the west door. Stone steps lead one down. The crypt is divided into compartments. There are graffiti and initials of prisoners on an ancient door which leans against a stone partition. Substantial strap hinges, though rusty, still remain on the door, in which there is a spy-hole at eye-level. The latest date carved on the door looks like 1823. A prison cell, indeed, and grim reminder of past ages. Ascending the stone steps, just before emerging into the chapel, one is brought back with a jerk to the 1990s by the sight of an up-to-date electricity fuse box and switchboard!

The Chapel is the responsibility of the Parish Church which sees to its upkeep and cleaning. It is good to note that Holy Communion is celebrated each Tuesday in the Chapel at 11 am.

Today it stands high and dry above the river, but still on a small island and integral with the old bridge. However, the course of the river has been diverted some yards to the south, leaving the four pointed arches and the chapel's foundations out of the water in normal conditions. The southern abutment has been strengthened and connected to the new modern-style bridge by a half arch. It seems a pity that some of the cutwaters of the old bridge have been removed. The northern end of the old bridge is still coincident with the old side-walk of the road, from which the chapel can be entered as well as from the south side. The lovely brownish-red stone from which the original bridge and chapel were built has been retained throughout the preservation and restorative work.

One cannot conclude one's remarks on Rotherham Bridge without quoting from Miss Dorothy Greene, FSA, in her account of the chapel of Our Lady on Rotherham Bridge:

> "As one stands today on the old Rotherham Bridge, gazing on the busy scene dominated now, as of yore, by the great church of All Saints, one's mind swings back, the hum of modern traffic fades and for a moment one sees again that 'fair Rotherham' which to our ancestors was a 'greate towne', sees again the sunlight fall softly on the

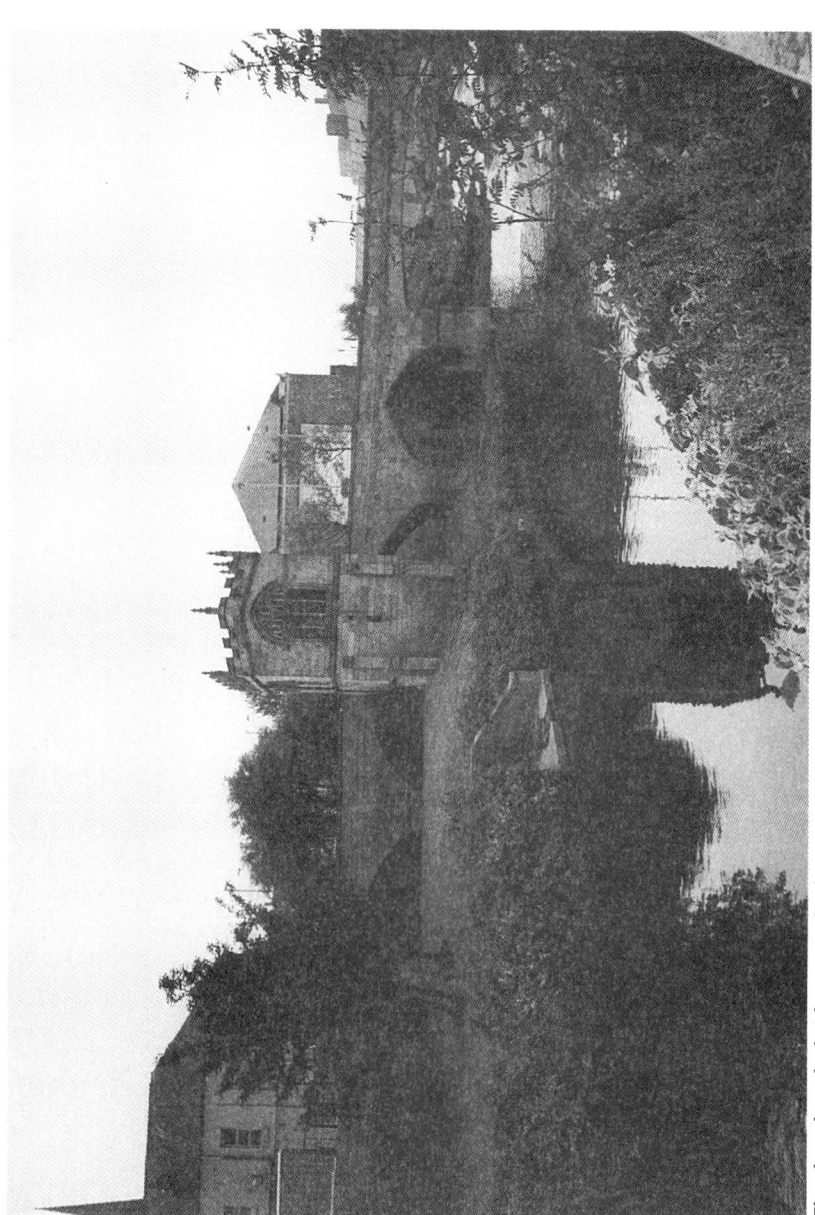

The chapel on the bridge at Rotherham. Note the new bridge on the right, showing the alteration in the course of the River Don from its original bed.

trees which line the Don; the sparkle of silver water, the flash of trout as he darts beneath the shadow of the bridge, and hears the sharp tramp of horses' feet as a procession, gay and vivid, winds over the narrow bridge. And what a procession time has led across that bridge! Flash of purple and gold as Thomas Rotherham rides by on his richly caparisoned mule; more somberly of hue as another Archbishop of York, Cardinal Wolsey, rides sadly by, a fallen and broken man in 1529; jingle of arms as the escort surrounding Mary, Queen of Scots, passes by, and the stern tramp of Ironsides, as Cromwell's men conduct her grandson, King Charles, to Rotherham on his journey to Whitehall and death. Later, softer things claim our attention, and a poetic figure leans upon the parapet as Ebenezer Elliott, the Corn Law Rhymer, watches the dappled trout and flash of birds in flight, and his contemporary, Ebenezer Rhodes, pauses on the bridge to watch the rays of the setting sun gild the great church, rising above the huddled roofs of houses and the stately elms which stand on the river's 'trembling edge'.

On that same bridge, in the Festival Year of 1951, we pause awhile to dream and then enter the little shrine where once again praise is raised to Almighty God."

Yorkshire is indeed blessed with so many bridges of beauty and romance. I hope that this book has whetted your appetite, and that you will have as much pleasure in seeking them out as I have done.